OTOLARYNGOLOGY RESEARCH ADVANCES

OBSTRUCTIVE AND CENTRAL SLEEP APNEA

Otolaryngology Research Advances

Additional books in this series can be found on Nova's website under the Series tab.

Additional e-books in this series can be found on Nova's website under the e-book tab.

OTOLARYNGOLOGY RESEARCH ADVANCES

OBSTRUCTIVE AND CENTRAL SLEEP APNEA

JOAN MCCORMICK
EDITOR

New York

Library of Congress Cataloging-in-Publication Data

ISBN: 978-1-63483-335-6

Published by Nova Science Publishers, Inc. † New York

Contents

Preface

The spectrum of sleep-disordered breathing ranges from primary snoring at one end to obstructive sleep apnea and central sleep apnea at the other end. The first chapter in this book provides current state of knowledge about the mechanisms of obstructive sleep apnea and central sleep apnea and reviews emerging therapies for these disorders. Furthermore, sleep apnea usually has multifactorial causes and affects multiple organic systems resulting in increased cardiovascular morbidity, disturbing sleep quality, metabolic balance, glucose and cholesterol levels, arterial hypertension and thus increasing cardiopulmonary and vascular morbidity. The second chapter summarizes the main findings in literature and provides a brief and concise differential diagnosis. The authors of the third chapter expose and discuss current evidence of neurosurgical conditions and their role in the genesis and progression of sleep apnea. They emphasize the adequate treatment and future perspectives. The following chapter examine the effect of obstructive sleep apnea syndrome (OSAS) on the eye. Different ophthalmologic disorders are associated with OSAS including floppy eyelid syndrome, retinal vein occlusion, and central serious retinopathy. The last chapter in this book is focused on QT dispersion in patients with obstructive sleep apnea, with increased QT dispersion potentially reflecting disturbed myocardial repolarization and predisposition to cardiac arrhythmias.

Chapter 1 – The spectrum of sleep-disordered breathing ranges from primary snoring at one end to obstructive sleep apnea and central sleep apnea at the other end. Obstructive sleep apnea and central sleep apnea have an impact on sleep quality and overall health. Repeated episodes of cessation or decrease in airflow and arousals from sleep occur during obstructive and central sleep apnea events. These episodes may lead to day time manifestations including, but not limited to, unrefreshed sleep, sleepiness, poor attention, hyperactivity, and fatigue. Unrecognized obstructive sleep apnea and central sleep apnea may cause cardiovascular, pulmonary, neurologic, metabolic, and neurocognitive morbidities. Better understanding the underlying pathophysiology of obstructive sleep apnea and central sleep apnea, and early diagnosis of sleep apnea and its consequences potentially prevent adverse effects on the individual. This article will provide current state of knowledge about the mechanisms of obstructive sleep apnea and central sleep apnea and review emerging therapies for these disorders.

Chapter 2 – Sleep apnea, characterized by repetitive cessation of breathing during sleep, has been reported to be prevalent in up to 30% of the general population and may be of obstructive or central origin. It has usually multifatorial causes and affects multiple organic systems resulting in increased cardiovascular morbidity, disturbing sleep quality, metabolic balance, glucose and cholesterol levels, arterial hypertension and thus increasing cardiopulmonary and vascular morbidity. Such complexity is generally assessed by several professionals, like clinical physicians, cardiologists, nutritionists, physical therapists, otorhinolaryngologists, pneumologists, endocrinologists and neurologists. Many neurological disorders, like epilepsy, dementia, neuromuscular affections, headache, multiple sclerosis and stroke may manifest or be characterized by specific sleep patterns, including sleep apnea. The authors summarize the main findings in literature and perform a brief and concise differential diagnosis.

Chapter 3 – Sleep apnea, characterized by repetitive cessation of breathing during sleep, has been reported to be prevalent in up to 30% of the general population and may be of obstructive or central origin. It has usually multifactorial causes and affects multiple organic systems like cardiovascular, sleep quality, metabolic balance, glucose and cholesterol levels, arterial hypertension and thus increasing cardiopulmonary and vascular morbidity. Such complexity is generally assessed by several professionals, like clinical physicians, cardiologists, nutritionists, physical therapists, otorhinolaryngologists, pneumologists, endocrinologists and neurologists. Nevertheless, increasing evidence points to the association of neurosurgical pathologies with sleep apnea, with potential reversibility after proper treatment. In this scenario, the authors expose and discuss current evidence of neurosurgical conditions and their role in the genesis and progression of sleep apnea. Additionally, they emphasize the adequate treatment and future perspectives.

Chapter 4 – Obstructive sleep apnea syndrome (OSAS) is defined by partial (hypopnea) or complete (apnea) intermittent episodes of upper airway collapse during sleep. The hypoxia resulting from these repetitive episodes leads to oxidative stress, sympathetic activation, endothelial dysfunction, systemic inflammation, and metabolic abnormalities. These pathophysiologic mechanisms are the source of many systemic diseases, such as blood and pulmonary hypertension, insulin resistance, metabolic syndrome, arrhythmia, myocardial infarction, congestive heart failure, and stroke. OSAS affects approximately 24% of men and 9% of women in the general population, and its prevalence increases with age. Different ophthalmologic disorders are also associated with OSAS: floppy eyelid syndrome, retinal vein occlusion, primary open angle glaucoma, normal-tension glaucoma, papilledema, non-ischemic anterior optic neuropathy, and central serous retinopathy. Changes in the optic nerve head (ONH) and retinal nerve fiber layer (RNFL) thickness in patients with OSAS have been a topic of controversy in recent years. Some studies have hypothesized that the hypoxia resulting from apnea-hypopnea episodes could compromise ONH vascularization. This condition may produce retinal ganglion cell damage and, consequently, reduce RFNL thickness. Some investigators report that OSAS and its severity could be related to decreased RNFL thickness or reduced retinal sensitivity measured with standard automated perimetry. On the other hand, other studies found no evidence of a correlation between OSAS and RFNL thickness loss. Different study designs, methodology, inclusion and exclusion criteria, age, and level of OSAS make it difficult to compare the results among several studies.

Thus, the structural and functional changes in the retina and optic disc due to OSAS remain unclear. Further prospective longitudinal studies are needed to elucidate the effect of OSAS on the eye.

Chapter 5 – Exaggerated dispersion of repolarization is likely to play a role in both the initiation and the maintenance of malignant ventricular arrhythmias. Inter-lead QT interval differences within a 12-lead ECG termed "QT dispersion" may reflect regional differences in myocardial refractoriness. QT dispersion is simply defined as the difference between the longest (QTmax) and the shortest (QTmin) QT intervals within a 12-lead ECG. Since the QT interval on its own may vary according to the heart rate, it may be corrected using Bazett's formula ($QT/\sqrt{RR}$) to give rise to QTc intervals, and the difference between QTcmax and QTcmin is the QTc dispersion (heart rate-corrected QT dispersion, QTcd). It has been supposed that one of the causes of the disturbed repolarization might be linked with autonomic imbalance, in that a decreased parasympathetic innervation exposes the heart to unopposed stimulation by sympathetic nerves. This assuming, abnormal QT dispersion may be related to obstructive sleep apnea syndrome (OSAS). A meta-analysis encompassing 222 patients with diagnosed OSAS and 182 control subjects found higher values of QT dispersion in OSAS patients. Another finding was more prominent increase in QT dispersion in the female OSAS patients. The reasons may be significantly longer values of QTd and QTcd found in healthy men. These normally higher values may explain why the OSAS in male patients resulted in less effect compared with women. Increased QT dispersion in OSAS patients may reflect disturbed myocardial repolarization and predispose to cardiac arrhythmias.

In: Obstructive and Central Sleep Apnea
Editor: Joan McCormick

ISBN: 978-1-63483-335-6

Chapter 1

Management of Obstructive and Central Sleep Apnea

Seckin O. Ulualp [*]
Department of Otolaryngology: Head and Neck Surgery,
University of Texas Southwestern Medical Center,
Dallas, TX, US

Abstract

The spectrum of sleep-disordered breathing ranges from primary snoring at one end to obstructive sleep apnea and central sleep apnea at the other end. Obstructive sleep apnea and central sleep apnea have an impact on sleep quality and overall health. Repeated episodes of cessation or decrease in airflow and arousals from sleep occur during obstructive and central sleep apnea events. These episodes may lead to day time manifestations including, but not limited to, unrefreshed sleep, sleepiness, poor attention, hyperactivity, and fatigue. Unrecognized obstructive sleep apnea and central sleep apnea may cause cardiovascular, pulmonary, neurologic, metabolic, and neurocognitive morbidities. Better understanding the underlying pathophysiology of obstructive sleep apnea

[*] Send correspondence to: Seckin O. Ulualp, MD, Department of Otolaryngology-Head and Neck Surgery, University of Texas Southwestern Medical Center, 5323 Harry Hines Blvd, Dallas, Texas, 75390-9035. Phone: (214) 456-2905. Fax: (214) 648-9122. E-mail: seckin.ulualp@utsouthwestern.edu.

and central sleep apnea, and early diagnosis of sleep apnea and its consequences potentially prevent adverse effects on the individual. This article will provide current state of knowledge about the mechanisms of obstructive sleep apnea and central sleep apnea and review emerging therapies for these disorders.

Keywords: Snoring, obstructive sleep apnea, central sleep apnea

Introduction

Sleep is critical for maintaining health and satisfactory quality of life in adults and children. Sleep disorders lead to decreased productivity and increased use of health care services [1]. It is estimated that 50-70 million individuals in United States are affected by sleep problems [1]. Early recognition and treatment of sleep disorders potentially prevents medical problems associated with sleep disordered breathing.

Sleep-related breathing disorder encompasses a range of conditions, including central sleep apnea, obstructive sleep apnea, upper airway resistance syndrome, and sleep-related hypoventilation or hypoxemic syndromes. The impact of obstructive and central sleep apnea on sleep quality and overall health has been widely documented. Repeated episodes of cessation or decrease in airflow and arousals from sleep occur during obstructive and central sleep apnea events. These episodes may lead to day time manifestations including, but not limited to, unrefreshed sleep, sleepiness, poor attention, hyperactivity, and fatigue. Furthermore, individuals suffering from obstructive sleep apnea or central sleep apnea have a higher risk for cardiovascular, pulmonary, neurologic, metabolic, and neurocognitive morbidities. Better understanding the underlying pathophysiology of obstructive sleep apnea and central sleep apnea, and early diagnosis of sleep apnea and its consequences potentially prevent adverse effects on the individual. This article will provide current state of knowledge about the mechanisms of obstructive sleep apnea and central sleep apnea and review emerging therapies for these disorders.

Pathogenesis

Obstructive Sleep Apnea

Collapse of the upper airway may trigger hypopneas, apneas, hypoventilation, causing obstructive sleep apnea. Decreased tonic activation of upper airway dilator musculature during sleep produces increased airway compliance and an enhanced collapsibility. Impaired compensatory activation of upper airway dilator musculature may lead to obstructive sleep apnea.

The length, width and collapsibility of the upper airway influence the air flow. Abnormalities of bony and soft tissue framework of the upper airway structures such as the internal and external nasal valves, nasal turbinates, nasal septum, cervical vertebrae, adenoid, soft palate, tonsillar pillars, tonsils, uvula, soft palate, pharyngeal fat pad and mucosa, pharyngeal muscles, tongue, lingual tonsils, epiglottis, maxilla, mandible, and hyoid alter the mechanics of the upper airway. The stability of the upper airway is also impaired due to changes in control of respiratory motor output, ventilatory control mechanisms, levels of consciousness, upper airway reflexes, peripheral nervous system mechanisms, and body position [2]. Severe abnormalities of the upper airway framework may progress to obstructive sleep apnea during sleep. Mildly collapsible upper airway may lead to obstructive sleep apnea in the presence of unstable central respiratory motor output.

Multi-site upper airway obstruction has been documented in patients with obstructive sleep apnea. Nasal obstruction increases airway resistance causing pharyngeal collapse, reduced muscular tone, and increased surface tension [3-6].

The upper airway configuration in obesity is characterized by increased fat distribution around the neck and displacement of lateral pharyngeal walls. Constricted airway in obesity contributes to obstructive sleep apnea [7]. Central ventilatory sensitivity in obesity originates from leptin and other cytokines [8, 9]. Abnormal shape, size and location of the mandible or maxilla may cause obstructive sleep apnea due to soft tissue impingement of the airway [10, 11]. Other sites of airway obstruction includes enlarged adenoid, tonsils or tongue, thickened lateral pharyngeal walls, displaced soft palate, and inferiorly located hyoid [12-21]. Body positioning contributes to obstructive sleep apnea by changing the airway size. Positioning from sitting to supine decreases airway size [22]. Variety of the mechanisms of obstructive sleep apnea, underlines the importance of the identification of obstruction sites and individualized treatment options.

Central Sleep Apnea

Central sleep apnea is characterized by repeated episodes of apnea associated with the temporary cessation of ventilatory effort. The ventilatory drive during sleep is controlled by complex interactions amongst the chemoreceptors, intrapulmonary receptors, cerebral cortex, and brainstem mechanisms [23, 24]. Alterations in the ventilator drive may cause central sleep apnea.

To date central sleep apnea has been categorized as complex central sleep apnea, idiopathic central sleep apnea, sleep transition apnea, and central sleep apnea. Central sleep apnea may occur physiologically, idiopathically, or in association with other disorders. Central apnea has been predominantly documented in patients with congestive heart failure, cerebrovascular disease, acromegaly, hypothyroidism, and high altitude [25-29]. Central sleep apnea may cause increased sympathetic neural activity 4, 5 affecting the cardiac function [3-32].

During sleep, decrease in metabolic demands requires altered alveolar ventilation causing changes in pH and CO_2 concentration [32-37]. In the absence of wakefulness stimulus, an enhanced bradypneic response to hypocarbia may occur [38]. When the carbon dioxide level is below the apnea threshold, a cessation of breathing may occur. Decreased neural respiratory drive and absence of muscular respiratory effort during sleep lead to central sleep apnea. Neural respiratory drive is restored upon augmentation of ventilation and reduced carbon dioxide levels when arousal from sleep occurs [39-42].

Diagnosis

High level of suspicion for obstructive sleep apnea and central sleep apnea is crucial for early identification and treatment. A careful sleep history including, but not limited to, snoring, daytime sleepiness, obesity, hypertension, or micro/retrognathia, is critical to screen or obstructive and central sleep apnea during a routine health maintenance evaluation or visit for a disorder associated with sleep disorders [46]. Identification of risk factors such as obesity (BMI > 35), congestive heart failure, atrial fibrillation, treatment of refractory hypertension, type 2 diabetes, nocturnal dysrhythmias, stroke, pulmonary hypertension, or preparation for bariatric surgery indicates the need for comprehensive sleep history. Comprehensive sleep history consists of assessment of snoring, pauses in breathing, apnea, episodes of gasping for air or choking at night, excessive sleepiness, feeling of tired in the morning, daytime somnolence, total sleep amount, nocturia, morning headaches, decreased concentration, memory loss, decreased libido, irritability, sleepiness severity by Epworth Sleepiness scale [43].

The physical examination of patient with suspected obstructive or central sleep apnea should include respiratory, cardiovascular and neurologic systems. Physical examination findings suggestive of obstructive sleep apnea include increased neck circumference, body mass index $\geq$ 30 kg/m^2, Modified Mallampati score of 3 or 4, micro/retrognathia, macroglossia, tonsillar hypertrophy, lingual tonsil hypertrophy, adenoid hypertrophy, elongated /enlarged uvula, high arched/narrow hard palate, or nasal abnormalities such as septal deviation, turbinate hypertrophy, internal/external nasal valve collapse [43].

The diagnosis of obstructive and sleep apnea can be established using polysomnography [44]. Patients with signs and symptoms suggestive of obstructive and central sleep apnea, should undergo sleep testing [44]. Polysomnogram is recommended to determine presence of obstructive sleep apnea in patients who will have bariatric surgery [43]. Home testing with portable monitors may be used to monitor response to positive airway pressure treatment and diagnose obstructive sleep apnea in patients who cannot perform in-laboratory polysomnogram. Follow-up polysomnogram or attended cardiorespiratory (type 3 portable monitoring) is needed for postsurgical assessment of moderate to severe obstructive sleep apnea and to ensure therapeutic benefit from oral appliance [44, 45]. Response to continuous positive airway pressure treatment should be monitored after substantial weight loss; i.e., such as 10% of body weight, substantial weight gain with return of symptoms, or insufficient clinical response [44].

Treatment

Obstructive Sleep Apnea

The patient with obstructive sleep apnea should be educated in the pathophysiology, risk factors, natural history and clinical consequences following review of polysomnogram findings [43]. Medical, behavioral, and surgical treatment options should be reviewed with the patient. Patients should be counseled on the role of weight loss, modification of risk factors such as avoiding alcohol and sedatives near bedtime, avoiding supine position, and risks associated with occupation and driving [43].

Non-surgical treatment options encompass positive airway pressure treatment, behavioral strategies, and oral appliances. Surgical options and adjunctive therapies are offered depending on the severity of the obstructive sleep apnea, compliance with positive airway pressure treatment, and airway abnormalities. Positive airway pressure treatment should be offered to all patients with obstructive sleep apnea. In effort to increase compliance with the use of positive airway pressure treatment, the patient should be educated about the function, care and maintenance of their equipment as well as benefits of treatment and potential problems. The usage of positive airway pressure treatment should be monitored with time meters [46].

Oral appliances, mandibular repositioning appliances, and tongue retaining devices decrease upper airway collapsibility and improve upper airway patency [47]. Patients with mild to moderate obstructive sleep apnea who are not candidates for positive airway pressure treatment may benefit from oral appliances [48]. After final adjustment of oral appliance, a polysomnogram or an attended cardiorespiratory sleep study should be obtained to confirm the benefit from the appliance [48].

Surgical treatment of obstructive sleep apnea begins with the counseling the patient on the surgical options, goals of treatment, successes rate, risks and benefits of the procedure, complications, alternative treatments and side effects [43]. Surgical procedure may be considered as a secondary treatment for patients who have unresolved obstructive sleep apnea despite use of positive airway pressure treatment and oral appliances.

Bariatric surgery, pharmacologic agents and oxygen therapy are adjunctive therapies for obstructive sleep apnea. Bariatric surgery can be considered as an adjunct treatment for obese patients with obstructive sleep apnea. Bariatric surgery is indicated in individuals with a body mass index $\geq$

40 kg/m^2 or body mass index $\geq$ 35 kg/m^2 with comorbidities [49]. Topical nasal steroids can be used in the presence of concurrent rhinitis [50]. Modafinil is recommended for treatment of residual excessive daytime sleepiness despite positive airway pressure treatment [50].

Central Sleep Apnea

Treatment options for central sleep apnea encompass to mechanical devices, respiratory stimulant drugs and supplemental O2 and CO2. Nasal continuous positive airway pressure (CPAP) therapy prevents pharyngeal narrowing and hence alleviating the ventilatory overshoot and perpetuation of ventilatory instability [51-53]. Nasal noninvasive positive pressure ventilation (NIPPV) restores alveolar hypoventilation and is used to treat central sleep apnea secondary to hypoventilation caused by neuromuscular or chest wall abnormalities [54].

The role of respiratory stimulant drugs has been limited to small studies supporting the use of acetazolamide and theophylline [55]. To date, no controlled clinical trials have been conducted to document the outcomes respiratory stimulant drugs in the treatment of central sleep apnea. Central sleep apnea associated with congestive heart failure, hypothyroidism, or acromegaly may be treated with, optimization of medical therapy. Supplemental oxygen may alleviate central sleep apnea by the suppression of the hypercapnic and the hypoxic ventilatory drives [56].

Conclusion

The impact of obstructive and central sleep apnea on sleep quality and overall health has been widely documented. Repeated episodes of cessation or decrease in airflow and arousals from sleep occur during obstructive and central sleep apnea events. These episodes may lead to day time manifestations including, but not limited to, unrefreshed sleep, sleepiness, poor attention, hyperactivity, and fatigue. Furthermore, individuals suffering from obstructive sleep apnea or central sleep apnea have a higher risk for cardiovascular, pulmonary, neurologic, metabolic, and neurocognitive morbidities. Early identification and treatment of obstructive and central sleep apnea provides significant relief for individuals, prevents complications and reduces overall health care costs.

Patients at high risk for obstructive and central sleep apnea need to have polysomnogram to confirm the diagnosis and to determine the severity of the disease. The treatment of obstructive and sleep apnea includes medical, behavioral and surgical options presented in a multidisciplinary setting and therapeutic approaches should be individualized to the severity of apnea and the patient's desire.

References

[1] Institute of Medicine. *Sleep disorders and sleep deprivation: An unmet* public health problem. Washington, DC: The National Academies Press; 2006. Available at http://www.iom.edu/cms/3740/23160/33668.aspx.

[2] Woodson B. T., Franco R. Physiology of sleep disordered breathing. *Otolaryngol Clin North Am*. 2007; 40(4):691-711.

[3] Young, L. Finn and H. Kim, Nasal obstruction as a risk factor for sleep-disordered breathing, *Allergy Clin Immunol* 1997; 99,757-762.

[4] Meurice J., Marc I., Carrier G. et al., Effects of mouth opening on upper airway collapsibility in normal sleeping subjects. *Am J Respir Crit Care* Med 1996; 153:255-259.

[5] Schwab R. J., Gefter W. B., Hoffman E. A. et al., Dynamic upper airway imaging during respiration in normal subjects and patients with sleep disordered breathing. *Am Rev Respir Dis* 1993; 148:1385-1400.

[6] Schwab R. J., Parirstein M., Pierson R. et al., Identification of upper airway anatomic risk factors for obstructive sleep apnea with volumetric MRI. *Am J Respir Crit Care Med* 2003; 167:1176-1180.

[7] Bradley T. D., Brown I. G., Grossman R. F. et al., Pharyngeal size in snorers, nonsnorers, and patients with obstructive sleep apnea. *N Engl J Med*. 1986; 315(21):1327-31.

[8] Kryger M., Felipe L., Holder D. et al., The sleep deprivation syndrome of the obese patient- a problem of periodic nocturnal upper airway obstruction. *Am J Med* 1974; 56: 531-9.

[9] Mortimore I., Marshall I., Wraith P. et al., Neck and total body fat deposition in non-obese and obese patients with obstructive sleep apnea compared with that in control subjects. *Am J Respir Crit Care Med* 1998; 157:280-3.

[10] Ferguson K. A., Ono T., Lowe A. A. et al., The relationship between obesity and craniofacial structure in obstructive sleep apnea. *Chest* 1995; 108: 375-38.

[11] Watanabe T., Isono S., Tanaka A. et al., Contribution of body habitus and craniofacial characteristics to segmental closing pressures of the passive pharynx in patients with sleep-disordered breathing. *Am J Respir Crit Care Med* 2002; 165: 260-265.

[12] Young J. W. and McDonald J. P. An investigation into the relationship between the severity of obstructive sleep apnoea/hypopnoea syndrome and the vertical position of the hyoid bone. *Surgeon* 2: 145-151, 2004.

[13] Riha R. L., Brander P., Vennelle M. et al., A cephalometric comparison of patients with sleep apnea/hypopnea syndrome and their siblings. *Sleep* 2005; 28: 315-320.

[14] Schwab R. J., Pasirstein M., Pierson R. et al., Identification of upper airway anatomic risk factors for obstructive sleep apnea with volumetric magnetic resonance imaging. *Am J Respir Crit Care Med* 2003; 168: 522-530.

[15] Schellenberg J. B., Maislin G. and Schwab R. J. Physical findings and the risk for obstructive sleep apnea. The importance of oropharyngeal structures. *Am J Respir Crit Care Med* 2000; 162:740-748.

[16] Schwab R. J., Gupta K. B., Gefter W. B. et al., Upper airway and soft tissue anatomy in normal subjects and patients with sleep-disordered breathing. Significance of the lateral pharyngeal walls. *Am J Respir Crit Care Med* 1995; 152:1673-1689.

[17] Schwab R. J., Pasirstein M., Pierson R. et al., Identification of upper airway anatomic risk factors for obstructive sleep apnea with volumetric magnetic resonance imaging. *Am J Respir Crit Care Med* 2003;168: 522-530.

[18] Greenfeld M., Tauman R., De Rowe A. et al., Obstructive sleep apnea syndrome due to adenotonsillar hypertrophy in infants. *Int J Pediatr Otorhinolaryngol* 2003; 67: 1055-1060.

[19] Bradley T. D., Rutherford R., Grossman R. F. et al., Role of daytime hypoxemia in the pathogenesis of right heart failure in the obstructive sleep apnea syndrome. *Am Rev Respir Dis* 1985; 131: 835-839.

[20] Ingman T., Nieminen T. and Hurmerinta K. Cephalometric comparison of pharyngeal changes in subjects with upper airway resistance syndrome or obstructive sleep apnoea in upright and supine positions. *Eur J Orthod* 2004; 26: 321-326.

[21] Stauffer J. L., Buick M. K., Bixler E. O. et al., Morphology of the uvula in obstructive sleep apnea. *Am Rev Respir Dis* 1989; 140: 724-728.

[22] Beaumont M., Fodil R., Isabey D. et al., Gravity effects on upper airway area and lung volumes during parabolic flight. *J Appl Physiol* 1998; 84(5):1639-45.

[23] Phillipson E. A. Control of breathing during sleep. *Am Rev Respir Dis* 1978; 118: 909-939.

[24] Eckert D. J., Jordan A. S., Merchia P., Malhotra A. Central sleep apnea: pathophysiology and treatment. *Chest* 2007; 131: 595-607.

[25] Buckle P., Millar T., Kryger M. The effect of short-term nasal CPAP on Cheyne-Stokes respiration in congestive heart failure. *Chest* 1992; 102: 31-35.

[26] Naughton M. T., Benard D. C., Rutherford R., Bradley T. D. Effect of continuous positive airway pressure on central sleep apnea and nocturnal PCO2 in heart failure, *American Journal of Respiratory and Critical Care Medicine* 1994;150:1598-1604, 1994.

[27] Willson G. N., Wilcox I., Piper A. J. et al., Noninvasive pressure preset ventilation for the treatment of Cheyne-Stokes respiration during sleep. *European Respiratory Journal* 2001; 17; 1250-1257.

[28] Teschler H., D¨ohring J., Wang Y. M., Berthon-Jones M. Adaptive pressure support servo-ventilation: a novel treatment for Cheyne-Stokes respiration in heart failure. *American Journal of Respiratory and Critical Care Medicine* 2001; 164:614-619.

[29] Johnson K. G., Johnson D. C. Bilevel positive airway pressure worsens central apneas during sleep. *Chest* 2005; 128:2141-2150.

[30] Kasai T. Sleep apnea and heart failure. *J Cardiol* 2012; 60: 78-85.

[31] Leung R. S., Diep T. M., Bowman M. E., Lorenzi-Filho G., Bradley T. D. Provocation of ventricular ectopy by cheyne-stokes respiration in patients with heart failure. *Sleep* 2004; 27: 1337-1343.

[32] Johansson P., Alehagen U., Svanborg E., Dahlstrom U., Brostrom A. Sleep disordered breathing in an elderly community-living population: relationship to cardiac function, insomnia symptoms and daytime sleepiness. *Sleep Med* 2009; 10:1005-1011.

[33] Douglas N. J., White D. P., Weil J. V. et al., Hypoxic ventilator response decreases during sleep in normal men. *Am Rev Respir Dis* 1982; 125(3): 286-289.

[34] Douglas N, J., White D. P., Weil J. V., Pickett C. K., Zwillich C. W. Hypercapnic ventilatory response in sleeping adults. *Am Rev Respir Dis* 1982; 126: 758-762.

[35] White D. P., Douglas N. J., Pickett C. K., Weil J. V., Zwillich C. W. Hypoxic ventilatory response during sleep in normal premenopausal women. *Am Rev Respir Dis* 1982; 126: 530-533.

[36] Wiegand L., Zwillich C. W., White D. P. Sleep and the ventilator response to resistive loading in normal men. *J Appl Physiol* 1988; 64: 1186-1195.

[37] Joseph V., Pequignot J. M., Van Reeth O. Neurochemical perspectives on the control of breathing during sleep. *Respir Physiol Neurobiol* 2002; 130:253-263.

[38] Krimsky W. R., Leiter J. C., Physiology of breathing and respiratory control during sleep. *Semin Respir Crit Care Med* 2005; 26: 5-12.

[39] Eckert D. J., Jordan A. S., Merchia P., Malhotra A. Central sleep apnea: pathophysiology and treatment. *Chest* 2007; 131:595-607.

[40] Malhotra A., Owens R. L. What is central sleep apnea? *Respir Care* 2010; 55:1168-1178.

[41] Kryger M. H., Roth T., Dement W. C. *Principles and Practice of Sleep Medicine*. 2nd ed. Philadelphia, PA: Saunders; 1994.

[42] Eckert D. J., Malhotra A., Jordan A. S. Mechanisms of apnea. *Prog Cardiovasc Dis*. 2009; 51:313-323.

[43] Epstein L. J., Kristo D., Strollo P. J. Jr. et al., Adult Obstructive Sleep Apnea Task Force of the American Academy of Sleep Medicine. Clinical guideline for the evaluation, management and long-term care of obstructive sleep apnea in adults. *J Clin Sleep Med*. 2009; 5(3):263-76.

[44] Kushida C. A., Littner M. R., Morgenthaler T. et al., Practice parameters for the indications for polysomnography and related procedures: An update for 2005. *Sleep* 2005; 28:499-521.

[45] Basner R. C., Ringler J., Schwartzstein R. M. et al., Phasic electromyographic activity of the genioglossus increases in normal during slow-wave sleep. *Respir Physiol* 1991; 83: 189-200.

[46] Kushida C. A., Littner M. R., Hirshkowitz M. et al., Practice parameters for the use of continuous and bilevel positive airway pressure devices to treat adult patients with sleep-related breathing disorders. *Sleep* 2006; 29:375-80.

[47] Ferguson K. A., Cartwright R., Rogers R. et al., Oral appliances for snoring and obstructive sleep apnea: a review. *Sleep* 2006; 29:244-62.

[48] Kushida C. A., Morgenthaler T. I., Littner M. R. et al., Practice parameters for the treatment of snoring and Obstructive Sleep Apnea with oral appliances: an update for 2005. *Sleep* 2006; 29:240-3.

[49] SAGES Guidelines Committee. *Guidelines for clinical application of laparoscopic bariatric surgery*: Society of American Gastrointestinal and Endoscopic Surgeons; 2008.

[50] Morgenthaler T. I., Kapen S., Lee-Chiong T. et al., Practice parameters for the medical therapy of obstructive sleep apnea. *Sleep* 2006; 29: 1031-5.

[51] Mehra R., Stone K. L., Blackwell T., Israel S. A., Dam T. T., Stefanick ML, et al., Prevalence and correlates of sleep-disordered breathing in older men: Osteoporotic Fractures in Men Sleep Study. Osteoporotic Fractures in Men Study. *J Am Geriatr Soc* 2007; 55:1356-64.

[52] Issa F. G., Sullivan C. E. Reversal of central sleep apnoea using nasal CPAP. *Chest* 1986; 90: 165-71.

[53] Hoffstein V., Slutsky A. S. Central sleep apnoea reversed by continuous positive airway pressure. *Am Rev Respir Dis* 1987; 135:1210-2.

[54] Guilleminault C., Stoohs R., Schnieder H., Podszus T., Peter J. H., von Wichert P. Central alveolar hypoventilation and sleep: treatment by intermittent positive-pressure ventilation through nasal mask in an adult. *Chest* 1989; 96:1210-2.

[55] Hudgel D. W., Thanakitcharu S. Pharmacologic treatment of sleep-disordered breathing. *Am J Respir Crit Care Med* 1998; 158:691-9.

[56] Chowdhuri S., Badr S. Central sleep apnoea. *Indian J Med Res* 2010; 131:150-164.

In: Obstructive and Central Sleep Apnea
Editor: Joan McCormick
ISBN: 978-1-63483-335-6

Chapter 2

Specific Neurological Disorders and Sleep Disturbances

K. A. Norremose[1] and M. F. Oliveira[2,*]
[1]Neurology Service, Santa Paula Hospital, São Paulo, Brazil
[2]Department of Neurosurgery, Hospital do Servidor Público Estadual de São Paulo, São Paulo, Brazil

Abstract

Sleep apnea, characterized by repetitive cessation of breathing during sleep, has been reported to be prevalent in up to 30% of the general population and may be of obstructive or central origin. It has usually multifatorial causes and affects multiple organic systems resulting in increased cardiovascular morbidity, disturbing sleep quality, metabolic balance, glucose and cholesterol levels, arterial hypertension and thus increasing cardiopulmonary and vascular morbidity. Such complexity is generally assessed by several professionals, like clinical physicians, cardiologists, nutritionists, physical therapists, otorhinolaryngologists, pneumologists, endocrinologists and neurologists. Many neurological disorders, like epilepsy, dementia, neuromuscular affections, headache, multiple sclerosis and stroke may manifest or be characterized by specific

* Corresponding author: Matheus Fernandes de Oliveira. Av. Pedro de Toledo, 1800 – Vila Clementino, São Paulo – São Paulo – Brazil. E-mail: mafernoliv@yahoo.com.br.

sleep patterns, including sleep apnea. We summarize the main findings in literature and perform a brief and concise differential diagnosis.

Keywords: Sleep apnea, neurology, differential diagnosis, treatment

1. Introduction

Sleep apnea syndrome (SAS) is considered a sleep-related respiratory disorder, characterized by repetitive episodes of complete (apnea) or partial (hypopnea) low airflow during sleep [1, 2, 3, 4, 5].

The pathophysiology is multifactorial, leading to a chronic recurrent state of intermittent hypoxemia and reoxygenation during sleep, maintaining a state of oxidative stress, which seems to be the key to the pathophysiological manifestations, and is associated with the development of a number of high morbidity-mortality systematic complications, such as obesity, type 2 diabetes, metabolic syndrome, and cardiovascular and neuropsychological diseases [6, 7, 8, 9, 10].

SAS has been reported to be prevalent in 9–28% of the general population and is usually divided in two subtypes: central sleep apnea and obstructive sleep apnea [1, 2, 3, 7, 9, 14].

In central subtype, disorders in the respiratory centers act contributing to hypoventilation. In obstructive subtype, several anatomical and physiological disorders generate partial or complete obstruction of upper airways [1, 2, 3, 7, 9, 14].

Obstructive sleep apnea (OSA) usually happens in men and middle aged subjects, is related to snoring and the fragmentation of sleep exacerbate decrease in occupational performance. Episodes are worsened by sedatives and alcohol [6, 7, 8, 9, 10].

Central sleep apnea results from impairment of central respiratory control. They are responsible for less than 10% of apnea cases. There is not a clear link with obesity and snoring, like in OSA [6, 7, 8, 9, 10].

Any anatomical, physiological or pathological disturbance in ascending reticular activating system and its relations with thalamus and cortex may be causes for central sleep apnea, like poliomyelitis, tumors, infections, ischaemias, autonomic neuropathies and many other disorders [6, 7, 8, 9, 10].

Due to multiple putative mechanisms involved, multidisciplinary evaluation is mandatory. Support performed by clinicians, cardiologists, nutritionists, physical therapists, pneumologists, endocrinologists, otorhynolaringologysts and neurologists are often indicated. In specific cases, a craniofacial surgeon may also be consulted.

Neurological Conditions and Sleep Disturbances

1. Stroke

Sleep disturbances are well documented in many cerebral ischaemias syndromes, especially in paramedian thalamic and brainstem strokes [8, 9].

Brainstem is the main structure involved in genesis of sleep-wake cycles and thus several infarctions, mainly in posterior part of brainstem, may cause arousal problems [10, 11, 12, 13, 14].

Indeed, SAS is an independent risk factor for vascular morbidity and mortality. Apneas generate hypoxia and CO_2 retention, changing hemodynamic and autonomic responses during sleep [6, 7, 8, 9, 10].

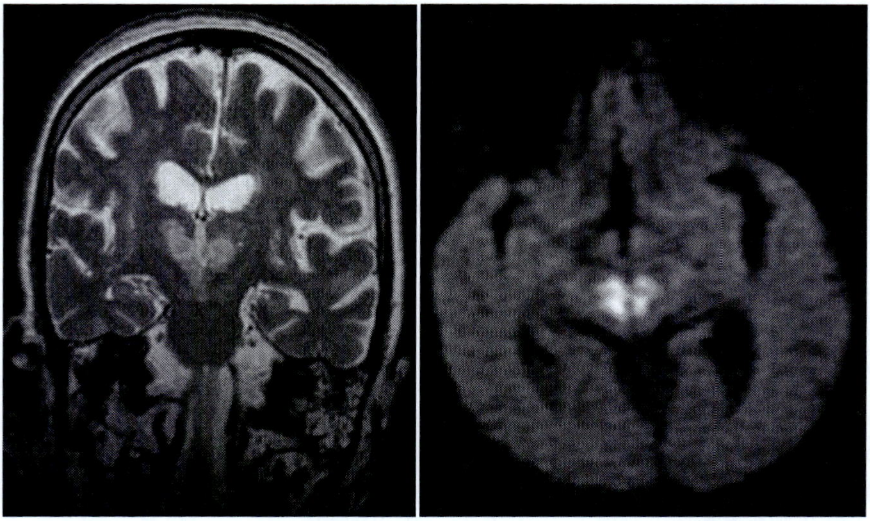

Figure 1. Paramedian thalamic infarctions (left) and brainstem stroke (right) are potential causes for sleep disturbances.

Some inflammatory factors, like cytokines, interleucines (IL-6), tumoral necrosis factor alfa and endothelins, may be involved in the genesis of associated arterial hypertension and intimal proliferation of vessels, associated with disorders of endothelium. Rapid intrathoracic pressure changes are also associated with changes in cardiac function and perfusion of neuronal tissue [11, 12, 13, 14].

On the other hand, vascular lesions may impair respiratory centers and determine important changes in respiratory patterns [6, 7, 8, 9, 10].

50 to 70% of inward patients with stroke may experiment sleep apnea in some time of hospitalization. Obstructive sleep apnea is usually more frequent than central sleep apnea, and this is also true for cases after a stroke [6, 7, 8, 9, 10].

2. Epilepsy

There is somehow a reciprocal relationship between sleep and epilepsy. Sleep increases interictal activity and thus facilitates seizures.

Additionally, deprivation of sleep may cause seizures by increasing cortical excitability. There is probably a greater prevalence of apnea in epileptic patients, however such reports are scattered and real dimension may not be adequately assessed [1, 2, 3, 4, 15, 16, 17].

Sleep seizures should be differentiated from NREM and REM parassonias, nocturnal panic attacks, psychogenic dissociated states, hypnic jerks, drug-induced diskynecias [1, 2, 3, 4, 15, 16, 17].

It is important to recognize involvement of epilepsy and sleep apnea, once treatment of apnea should improve seizure control.

3. Degenerative Dementia

Sleep dysfunction with or without motor activity is increasingly reported in non reversible dementia. Alzheimer disease is the most common presentation, but other types include, Lewy Body disease, Parkinson Disease, progressive supranuclear palsy, Huntington disease, Creutzfeldt-Jakob disease and other less common [4, 5, 6, 17, 18, 19, 20].

Major sleep disturbances include imsonia, hypersomnia, disorders in circadian rhythm. Some factors are usually identified in the genesis of such alterations: physiological changes of ageing, status of apolipoprotein E, comorbid conditions [4, 5, 6, 17, 18, 19, 20].

In Alzheimer Disease, sleep alterations may happen early. Their sleep is fragmented, with several waking and sometimes staying awake in the night. A special condition called sundowning is typical and refers to agitation in the late hours of afternoon, before evening. Sleep apnea can be present in up to 40% of patients and with the worsening of symptoms, patients may become sleepy, with imsomnia and visual hallucinations [4, 5, 6, 17, 18, 19, 20].

In Parkinson Disease (PD), sleep dysfunction is present in almost all patients. Insomnia is typical, followed by motor abnormalities during sleep. Other typical findings include daytime hypersomnolence and sleep attacks, which may be accentuated by dopaminergic medications. Daytime sleepiness was also highlighted with PD patients, particularly with the advent of newer dopamine agonists and the report of 'sleep attacks' in association with this group of drugs. Patients with PD need to be cautioned about possible daytime sleepiness when they start dopamine agonists. The daytime sleepiness may be accompanied by severe REMBD (rapid eye movement behavioral disorders), nocturia, night-time pain caused by immobility, bradykinesia, sleep apnoea or restless legs – all these are reported in association with PD.

Early and prominent sleep disturbance is more likely to be associated with early cognitive impairment. A careful sleep history should be taken in all patients with PD and sleep symptoms monitored throughout the disease [5, 6, 17, 18, 19, 20]. Frontotemporal dementia is probably linked to sleep disturbances, but no reports have addressed adequately these points. Sleep apnea is more common in vascular dementia than Alzheimer [20].

Huntington's disease patients often have particularly fragmented sleep, with an increase in periodic limb movements, sleep apnoea and daytime sleepiness [20].

4. Neuromuscular Disorders

Poliomyelites is probably the icon of relationship between sleep disturbances and neurological disorders. In the pre immunization era, many patients were affected and in the advanced phase of disease presented with respiratory failure and preserved conscience. Several hospitals had artificial lungs known as iron lungs, which performed passive ventilation in patients with muscular deficits. Neuromuscular disorders affect respiration due to involvement of respiratory muscles and nerves [1, 2, 3, 4, 5].

Some respiratory symptoms may be present in the onset of neuromuscular diseases. Several respiratory symptoms are characteristic in Duchenne dystrophy, limb-girdle dystrophy, myotonic dystrophy and other typical disorders [6, 7, 8, 9, 10]. In polineuropathies, involvement of nerves like intercostals and phrenic may generate various degrees of breathlessness. Neuromuscular junctional disorders like botulism, myasthenia gravis and Lambert-Eaton syndrome course with general and respiratory fatigability, being potentially involved with sleep apnea [5, 19, 20].

A wide range of progressive neuromuscular disorders can cause progressive weakness of respiratory muscles. This can lead in turn to nocturnal hypoventilation and gradual progression to respiratory failure. Many patients with such diseases complain of fatigue and reduced exercise tolerance because of skeletal muscle weakness, so symptoms of nocturnal ventilation can be missed unless careful screening is carried out early in the illness [19, 20, 21, 25, 26]. Examples of diseases that commonly cause significant respiratory failure include motor neuron disease (MND), Duchenne muscular dystrophy and myasthenia gravis.

Restless Legs Syndrome

Restless legs syndrome (RLS) is common, affecting 5–10% of the population, with associations with iron deficiency, dialysis and pregnancy [5, 19, 20]. There is a family history in 50% of affected patients. It is characterized by unpleasant sensations deep within calves and thighs that cause the patient to move, and has a clear circadian pattern being worse in the evening and first half of the night [5, 19, 20]. These symptoms contrast with peripheral neuropathy where dysaesthesia is usually maximal within the feet and there is no circadian pattern to symptoms or relief with movement. The associated periodic limb movements of sleep can fragment sleep enough to cause daytime sleepiness. Tricyclic antidepressants, such as amitriptyline, can make RLS worse so should be avoided, but gabapentin, dopamine agonists, such as ropinirole and pramipexole, clonazepam and opiates all help symptoms. Iron replacement should be used for ferritin levels below 45 mg/dl [5, 19, 20].

5. Spinal Cord Disorders

Patients with poliomyelitis, amyothophic lateral sclerosis (ALS), spinal cord trauma, spinal cord tumors and spinal surgery may have sleep disturbances due to varied reasons. The most frequent symptom is hypersomnia, but imsomnia and apena may be present [5, 19, 20, 21, 22].

In postpolio syndrome, apnea may be specially common. This syndrome is characterized by increasing weakness of muscles previously affected in the acute phase of poliomyelitis. ALS is the most common motor neuron disease in adults and may also be a putative cause for sleep disturbances., generally associated with muscle weakness, and being characterized by apnea, hypopnea and hypoxemia [23, 24].

Cervical trauma and cervical spinal tumors may have similar sleep presentations.

6. Headache

Sleep disturbances and headache are, separately, two of the most common causes of health complaints. Not coincidentally, there is a strong relationship between such conditions. Headache may cause sleep disturbances and vice-versa. In cluster headache, for example, there is a strong association of REM sleep and headache. Many relations are also observed with chronic headache, migraine, hemicrania and other types of headache. There are anecdotal reports of improvement in headaches after treatment of obstructive sleep apnea with continuous positive air pressure (CPAP) [21].

There is a specific headache syndrome called hypnic headache syndrome, which is described in patients over 60 years old and characterized by awaking during sleep due to headache [21].

7. Others

Neurological disorders related to sleep disturbances are frequent and typical features, being causes and sometimes consequences [25, 26, 27, 28, 29]. Other neurological syndromes, like demyelinative disorders and autonomic failures may also be equally involved with sleep pattern. As a general rule, an adequate sleep pattern demands psychological stability and functional neurologic structures. Any impairment of such structures generate symptoms, often presenting as apnea, imsomnia or hypersomnia [25, 26, 27, 28, 29].

References

[1] Franco, C. M., Lima, A. M., Ataíde, L. Jr, Lins, O. G., Castro, C. M., Bezerra, A. A., de Oliveira, M. F., Oliveira, J. R. Obstructive sleep apnea severity correlates with cellular and plasma oxidative stress parameters and affective symptoms. *J. Mol. Neurosci.* 2012 Jun;47(2): 300-10. doi: 10.1007/s12031-012-9738-0.

[2] Cao, J., Feng, J., Li, L., Chen, B. Obstructive sleep apnea promotes cancer development and progression: a concise review. *Sleep Breath.* 2015 Feb. 3.

[3] Gadoth, N., Oksenberg, A. Corrigendum: Sleep and Sleep Disorders in Rare Hereditary Diseases: A Reminder for the Pediatrician, Pediatric and Adult Neurologist, General Practitioner, and Sleep Specialist. *Front. Neurol.* 2015 Jan. 26;6:6. eCollection 2015.

[4] Santamaria, J., Iranzo, A. Sleep disorders matter in neurology. *Lancet Neurol.* 2014 Jan;13(1):18-20. doi: 10.1016/S1474-4422(13)70273-4.

[5] Anderson, K. Sleep disturbance and neurological disease. *Clin. Med.* 2011 Jun;11(3):271-4.

[6] Billiard, M. Neurological diseases and sleep disorders: a mutual enlightment. *Rev. Neurol.* (Paris). 2008 Aug-Sep;164(8-9):625-6. doi: 10.1016/j.neurol.2008.07.001. Epub. 2008 Aug. 28.

[7] Culebras, A. Neurology of sleep. *Rev. Neurol. Dis.* 2011;8(3-4):e114-9.

[8] Ahn, S. H., Kim, J. H., Kim, D. U., Choo, I. S., Lee, H. J., Kim, H. W. Interaction between Sleep-Disordered Breathing and Acute Ischemic Stroke. *J. Clin. Neurol.* 2013 Jan;9(1):9-13.

[9] Alam, I., Lewis, K., Stephens, J. W., Baxter, J. N. Obesity, metabolic syndrome and sleep apnoea: all pro-inflammatory states. *Obes. Rev.* 2007 Mar;8(2):119-27.

[10] Zee, P. C., Badr, M. S., Kushida, C., Mullington, J. M., Pack, A. I., Parthasarathy, S., Redline, S., Szymusiak, R. S., Walsh, J. K., Watson, N. F. Strategic opportunities in sleep and circadian research: report of the Joint Task Force of the Sleep Research Society and American Academy of Sleep Medicine. *Sleep.* 2014 Feb. 1;37(2):219-27. doi: 10. 5665/sleep.3384.

[11] Yaggi, H. K., Cancato, J., Karen, W. N. Obstructive sleep apnea as a risk factor for stroke and death. *N. Engl. J. Med.* 2005;353:2034-41.

[12] McnNicholas, W. T., Bonsignore, M. R. the Management Committee of EU COST ACTION B26. Sleep apnea as independent risk factor for

cardiovascular disease: Current evidence, basic mechanisms and research priorities. *Eur. Respir. J.* 2007;29:156-78.

[13] Lee, W., Lee, S. A., Chung, Y. S., Kim, W. S. The Relation Between Apnea and Depressive Symptoms in Men with Severe Obstructive Sleep Apnea: Mediational Effects of Sleep Quality. *Lung*. 2015 Jan. 30.

[14] Ramos, A. R., Tarraf, W., Rundek, T., Redline, S., Wohlgemuth, W. K., Loredo, J. S., Sacco, R. L., Lee, D. J., Arens, R., Lazalde, P., Choca, J. P., Mosley, T. Jr, González, H. M. Obstructive sleep apnea and neurocognitive function in a Hispanic/Latino population. *Neurology*. 2015 Jan. 27;84(4):391-8. doi: 10.1212/WNL.0000000000001181. Epub. 2014 Dec. 24.

[15] Spira, A. P., Yager, C., Brandt, J., Smith, G. S., Zhou, Y., Mathur, A., Kumar, A., Brašić, J. R., Wong, D. F., Wu, M. N. Objectively Measured Sleep and β-amyloid Burden in Older Adults: A Pilot Study. *SAGE Open Med.* 2014 Aug. 12;2. doi: 10.1177/2050312114546520.

[16] Arnulf, I., Leu, S., Oudiette, D. Abnormal sleep and sleepiness in Parkinson's disease. *Curr. Opin. Neurol.* 2008 Aug;21(4):472-7.

[17] Happe, S., Trenkwalder, C. Movement disorders in sleep: Parkinson's disease and restless legs syndrome. *Biomed. Tech.* (Berl.). 2003 Mar;48 (3):62-7.

[18] Comella, C. L. Sleep disorders in Parkinson's disease: an overview. *Mov. Disord.* 2007 Sep;22 Suppl. 17:S367-73. doi: 10.1002/mds.21682.

[19] Culebras, A. Repercussion of sleep apnea in neurology. *Rev. Neurol.* 2003 Jan. 1-15;36(1):67-70.

[20] Yaffe, K., Falvey, C. M., Hoang, T. Connections between sleep and cognition in older adults. *Lancet Neurol.* 2014 Oct;13(10):1017-28. doi: 10.1016/S1474-4422(14)70172-3.

[21] Stark, C. D., Stark, R. J. Sleep and chronic daily headache. *Curr. Pain Headache Rep.* 2015 Jan;19(1):468. doi: 10.1007/s11916-014-0468-6.

[22] Bianchi, M. T., Alameddine, Y., Mojica, J. Apnea burden: efficacy versus effectiveness in patients using positive airway pressure. *Sleep Med.* 2014 Dec;15(12):1579-81. doi: 10.1016/j.sleep.2014.07.015. Epub. 2014 Sep. 17.

[23] Fariborz Rezaeitalab, Fatemeh Moharrari, Soheila Saberi, Hadi Asadpour, and Fariba Rezaeetalab. The correlation of anxiety and depression with obstructive sleep apnea syndrome. *J. Res. Med. Sci.* 2014 Mar; 19(3): 205-210.

[24] Akashiba, T., Kavahara, S., Akahoshi, T., Omori, C., Saitto, O., Majima, T., et al. Relationship between quality of life and mood or depression in

patients with severe obstructive sleep apnea syndrome. *Chest*. 2002;122: 861-5.

[25] Morimoto, S., Takahashi, T., Okaishi, K., Okuro, M., Nakahashi, T., Sakamado, D., et al. Sleep apnoea syndrome as a risk for mortality in elderly inpatients. *J. Inter. Med. Res*. 2012;40:601-11.

[26] Sharafkhaneh, A., Giray, N., Richardson, P., Young, T., Hirshkowitz, M. Association of Psychiatric disorders and sleep apnea in a large cohort. *Sleep*. 2005;28:1405-11.

[27] Marrie, R. A., Reider, N., Cohen, J., Trojano, M., Sorensen, P. S., Cutter, G., Reingold, S., Stuve, O. A systematic review of the incidence and prevalence of sleep disorders and seizure disorders in multiple sclerosis. *Mult. Scler*. 2014 Dec. 22. pii: 1352458514564486.

[28] Brass, S. D., Duquette, P., Proulx-Therrien, J., Auerbach, S. Sleep disorders in patients with multiple sclerosis. *Sleep Med. Rev*. 2010 Apr;14(2):121-9. doi: 10.1016/j.smrv.2009.07.005. Epub. 2009 Oct. 29.

[29] Barun, B. Pathophysiological background and clinical characteristics of sleep disorders in multiple sclerosis. *Clin. Neurol. Neurosurg*. 2013 Dec; 115 Suppl. 1:S82-5. doi: 10.1016/j.clineuro.2013.09.028.

In: Obstructive and Central Sleep Apnea
Editor: Joan McCormick
ISBN: 978-1-63483-335-6

Chapter 3

Neurosurgical Topics and Sleep Apnea

***M. F. Oliveira*[1,*], *K. A. Norremose*[2] *and F. C. G. Pinto*[3]**

[1]Department of Neurosurgery, Hospital do Servidor Público Estadual de São Paulo, São Paulo, Brazil
[2]Neurology Service, Santa Paula Hospital, São Paulo, Brazil
[3]Division of Functional Neurosurgery of the Institute of Psychiatry, Hospital das Clínicas, Universidade de São Paulo, São Paulo, Brazil

Abstract

Sleep apnea, characterized by repetitive cessation of breathing during sleep, has been reported to be prevalent in up to 30% of the general population and may be of obstructive or central origin. It has usually multifactorial causes and affects multiple organic systems like cardiovascular, sleep quality, metabolic balance, glucose and cholesterol levels, arterial hypertension and thus increasing cardiopulmonary and vascular morbidity. Such complexity is generally assessed by several professionals, like clinical physicians, cardiologists, nutritionists, physical therapists, otorhinolaryngologists, pneumologists,

* Corresponding author: Matheus Fernandes de Oliveira. Av. Pedro de Toledo, 1800 – Vila Clementino, São Paulo – São Paulo – Brazil. E-mail: mafernoliv@yahoo.com.br.

endocrinologists and neurologists. Nevertheless, increasing evidence points to the association of neurosurgical pathologies with sleep apnea, with potential reversibility after proper treatment. In this scenario, we expose and discuss current evidence of neurosurgical conditions and their role in the genesis and progression of sleep apnea. Additionally, we emphasize the adequate treatment and future perspectives.

Keywords: Sleep apnea, neurosurgery, diagnosis, treatment

Introduction

Sleep apnea syndrome (SAS) is considered a sleep-related respiratory disorder, characterized by repetitive episodes of complete (apnea) or partial (hypopnea) low airflow during sleep [1, 2, 3]. The pathophysiology is multifactorial, leading to a chronic recurrent state of intermittent hypoxemia and reoxygenation during sleep, maintaining a state of oxidative stress, which seems to be the key to the pathophysiological manifestations, and is associated with the development of a number of high morbidity-mortality systemic complications, such as obesity, type 2 diabetes, metabolic syndrome, and cardiovascular and neuropsychological diseases [1, 2, 3].

SAS has been reported to be prevalent in 9–28% of the general population and is usually divided in two subtypes: central sleep apnea and obstructive sleep apnea (the most frequent subbtype, accounting for approximately 80% of cases) [1, 2, 3]. In central subtype, disorders in the respiratory centers act contributing to hypoventilation. In obstructive subtype, several anatomical and physiological disorders generate partial or complete obstruction of upper airways [1, 2, 3].

Due to multiple putative mechanisms involved, multidisciplinary evaluation is mandatory. Support performed by clinicians, cardiologists, nutritionists, physical therapists, pneumologists, endocrinologists, otorhynolaringologysts and neurologists are often indicated. In specific cases, a craniofacial surgeon may also be consulted [1, 2, 3].

Increasing scientific evidence has established some relationship between SAS and uncommon but varied neurosurgical conditions. Elevations in intracranial pressure related to respiration, especially Cheyne-Stokes respiration, are well known and the association of increased intracranial pressure with sleep apnea is not new. It has already been shown that awake values for intracranial pressures (ICP) are pathologically elevated in patients with severe SAS. ICP increases further during sleep, especially NREM stages 2 to 3 and REM sleep related to the apneic episodes, and strong correlations between durations of apnea and ICP elevations.

Mechanisms involved are probably multiple, with the participation of cytokines, vasomotor and vasoplegic factors and activation of breathing centers. The role of obesity and vasculature resistence and complacency may also be very important.

We discuss in this chapter some important aspects concerning neurosurgery and sleep apnea.

Neurosurgical Conditions and Sleep Apnea

1. Hydrocephalus

Hydrocephalus is a condition characterized by dilated cerebrospinal fluid compartments [4, 5, 6, 7]. There are different classifications, but the most common divide hydrocephalus in communicant and obstructive; acute and chronic and congenital or acquired. As a final result, enlarged ventricles are generally associated with increasing of intracranial pressure. Thus, several reports have associated symptoms of SAS with hydrocephalus. On the other hand, normal pressure hydrocephalus is also associated with SAS [4, 5, 6, 7].

Normal pressure hydrocephalus (NPH) is caused by a disturbance of cerebrospinal fluid (CSF) circulation with normal CSF pressure. Although with mean intracranial pressure within normal limits, its qualitative analysis is characterized by Lundberg *B* waves with amplitude of up to 50 mmHg, especially at night, probably related to different sleep stages, apnea episodes and rhythmic alterations of cerebral blood flow. Thus, this high resistence and low complacency environment would promote hypoperfusional deficits and interstitial edema, being even associated with apneas and sleep disorders [8, 9, 10, 11, 12].

Although the classic triad of subcortical dementia, gait apraxia and urinary incontinence is the most common, there are several other clinical pictures, including tremor, apendicular ataxia, psychiatric manifestations like anxiety and psychosis and even oligosymptomatic cases [9, 10, 11, 12].

Central sleep apneas and obstructive sleep apneas may be potential targets in the treatment of hydrocephalus (Figure 1), once increasing reports have associated ventricular shunting with improvement of symptoms. However, larger and controlled studies are still needed. Additionally, NPH patients should have their sleep profiles routinely evaluated from the diagnosis to the post operative period, once this finding may be potentially more frequent than thought [11, 12].

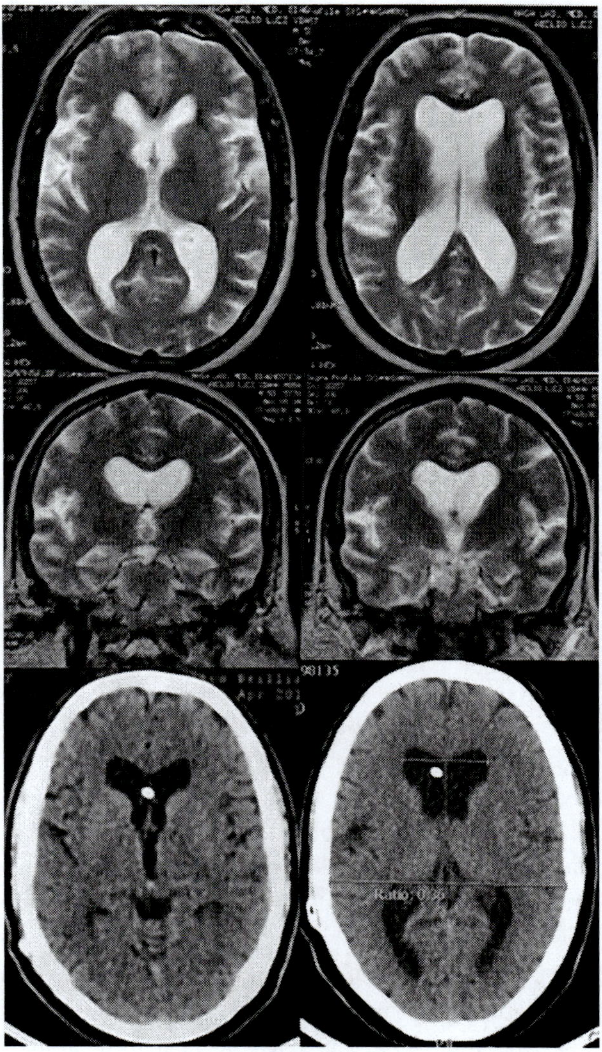

Figure 1. A subject of 62 years old with improvement of 70% in central sleep apnea after ventricular shunting for normal pressure hydrocephalus.

2. Craniocervical Disorders

2.1. Chiari Malformation

Craniovertebral junction malformations (CVJM) or Chiari malformation in adults, with or without syringomyelia and basilar invagination are mesodermic malformations usually characterized by different skull base craniometry and dimensions, producing neuronal dysfunction of the brainstem, cerebellum, cranial nerves, and upper spinal cord. The respiratory center and some of its afferent and efferent components can be altered in these diseases [13, 14, 15, 16]. There may be also compensatory changes in oral anatomy, with associated obstructive sleep apnea [13, 14, 15, 16].

Respiratory manifestations during sleep were studied with polysomnography in symptomatic patients with CVJM. Compared to healthy volunteers, they presented with more sleep disturbances (reports of snoring and apnea) than those in the control group. The apnea/hypopnea index values were higher in patients with CVJM than in the control group, being basilar invagination and syringomielia especially affected [13, 14, 15, 16, 17].

Among patients with Chiari malformation and CVJM, there is a clear relation of posterior fossa decompression surgery with improvement in number of respiratory events. There is also a lowered sleep fragmentation and enhanced sleep apnea index [17].

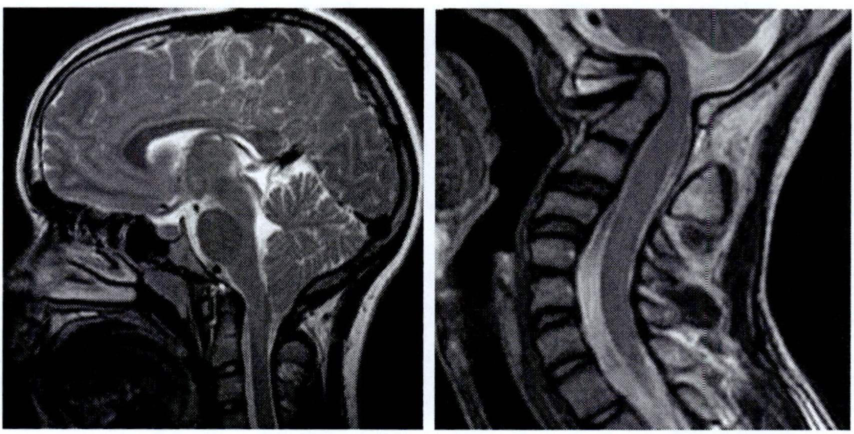

Figure 2. At left, a subject with Chiari malformation. At right, a case of basilar invagination.

2.2. Rheumatoid Arthritis

Rheumatoid arthritis (RA) is also known to be closely associated with increased cardiovascular risk and sudden death, and sleep apnea has been suggested to be a causal background. The prevalence of sleep apnea in RA patients may range 50%, sometimes affecting upper cervical spine and causing occipitocervical lesions, promoting associated symptomatology of central and obstructive apnea [13, 16, 17].

3. Cervical Disorders

3.1. Cervical Laminectomy

In 1994, Naim-ur-Rahman reported the first case of postoperative central sleep apnea following C3-C6 laminectomy, occurring right after surgery and associated with sphyncterial incontinence, that spontaneously recovered three weeks after onset [18, 19, 20].

Until now, other reports have also made such correlation, however strong causative reasons are lacking and predisposing factors are not known. There is no consensus in pathophysiology and risk groups. It is believed that severe cervical stenosis is associated with higher risk of sleep apnea postoperatively [21, 22].

3.2. Cervical Osteophytes

Following the same rationale, some cases of cervical osteophytes were related to sleep apnea.

Generally, osteophytes are asymptomatic and may lead to symptoms such as dysphagia, cough, dyspnea, and dysphonia. When large and causing important other symptoms, obstructive apnea may appear as a part of varied symptoms [20].

3.3. Cervical Tumors

Due to its relation with lower brainstem and cervical plexus, some reports of cervical tumors have pointed them as causes for sleep apnea. One of the most cited are encondromas [23].

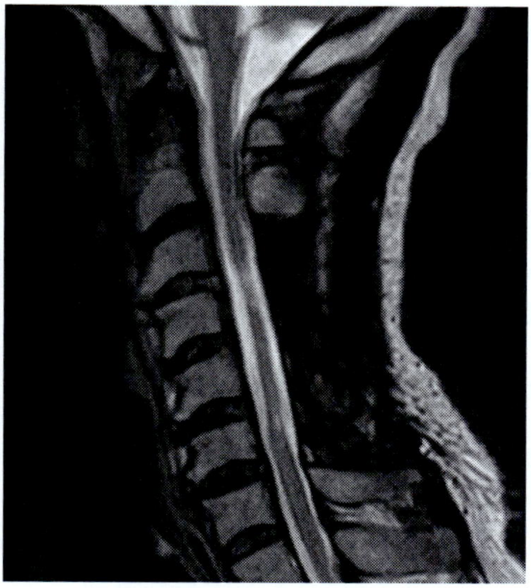

Figure 3. Typical post laminectomy aspect. Case with pre operative stenosis.

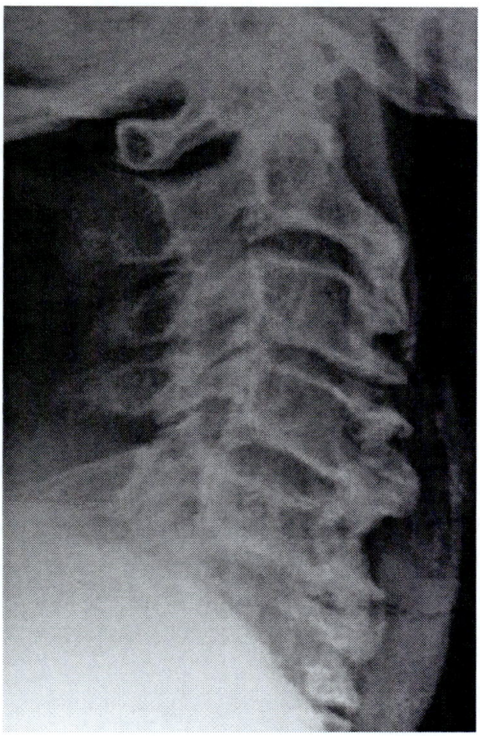

Figure 4. Important osteophytes generating compression of air column in trachea.

4. Pituitary Disorders

Sleep apnoea syndrome (SAS) is common in acromegaly and both diseases are independently associated with hypertension and insulin resistance contributing to increased morbidity and mortality [24].

5. Craniosynostosis

The association of Chiari malformation with syndromic craniosynostosis in children is well established. Central sleep apnea may subsequently occur. Some authors suggest posterior fossa decompression is an effective treatment modality for improving such symptoms [17, 18, 19].

6. Neoplasms

Neoplastic lesions involved in SAS may be origined in skull base, like chordomas and chondrossarcomas and encephaloceles; pharyngeal lipomas and growth hormone–secreting pituitary adenomas. Other rare lesions reported in association with SAS were encondromas, ependymomas, meningeomas and meduloblastoma [24].

Tumors of the brainstem and high cervical spinal cord may also be involved with obstructive and especially central sleep apnea, like lipomas of the mesencephalic tectum and rostral pons and brainstem gliomas [24].

7. Traumatic Brain Injury and Spinal Cord Injury

Traumatic brain injury is a common condition with high associated morbidity. From a mild to a severe traumatic brain injury, depending on the amount of lesion and status recovery, there may be sleep disturbances characterized by hypo or hypersomnolence, hypoxemia, and many degrees of sleep apnea. Similarly to what happens in cerebrovascular diseases, up to 60% of patients with traumatic brain injury may experience some kind of sleep disorder [25, 26].

Several symptoms follow traumatic brain injury (TBI), but patients commonly experience significant daytime sleepiness and can have sleep-wake reversal.

Levels of the neuropeptide hypocretin (undetectable in narcolepsy) have been shown to fall acutely following TBI and then gradually increase to normal levels.

For patients with persistent daytime sleepiness, agents such as modafinil or amantadine have been used with varying degrees of success [25, 26]. Similarly to brain injury, in spinal cord injury there may be association of depressive and anxiety states with lesion on upper spinal cord and lower brainstem, translating into high prevalence of sleep disorders, of 50% or above [25, 26].

Neurosurgical Targets for Treatment of Sleep Apnea

Therapeutic Targets

The advanced scientific dialogue of neurosurgery with sleep disorders have not only allowed the discovery of many "unknown" causes for sleep disorders, like cervical, intracranial and brainstem neurosurgical diseases, but has also allowed a different approach in their treatment, especially what concerns to functional neurosurgery and neuromodulation [27, 28, 29, 30].

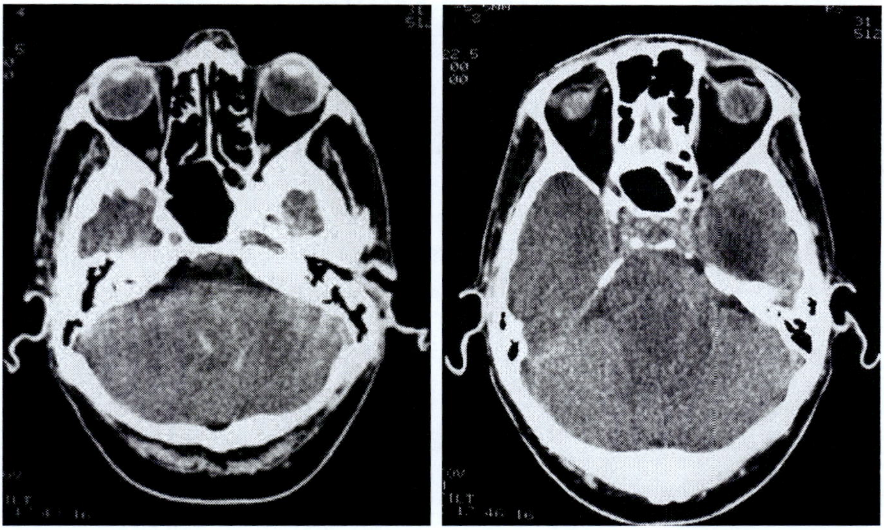

Figure 5. Post traumatic skull tomography, with image of lesions in brainstem.

Hypoglossal nerve stimulation is under investigation by multiple groups as a possible alternative therapy for obstructive sleep apnea. Targeted neurostimulation of the proximal hypoglossal nerve presents as a viable system approach that is far more versatile and physiologic and quite different than prior systems. Hypoglossal motoneurons are influenced by a variety of neuromodulators, some of which change dynamically across sleep-wake states to alter motoneuron excitability and responses to pharmacological manipulations [27, 28, 29, 30].

Significant reductions of snoring were reported after treatment with radiofrequency surgery of the tongue base in patients suffering from obstructive sleep apnea syndrome [27, 28, 29, 30].

The gold standard for the treatment of obstructive sleep apnea is continuous positive airway pressure (CPAP). It has been demonstrated that successful CPAP treatment improves systemic hypertension and prolongs survival. However, the clinical effectiveness of CPAP is often limited by low patient acceptance, poor tolerance, and suboptimal compliance. Therefore, non-CPAP alternatives for the treatment of sleep disordered breathing, such as oral appliance therapy with custom-made titratable mandibular advancement devices, surgery, or upper airway stimulation have gained growing interest [27, 28, 29, 30].

Conclusion

There is a clear and enlarging interface between sleep apnea and neurosurgical conditions. Physicians dealing with SAS must be aware of some uncommon causes for sleep disturbances. Those patients must be fully investigated, including nasopharyngeal endoscopy and neuroradiological images to exclude obstructive and neurosurgical lesions.

Additionally, neurosurgical community is facing functional targets to treat sleep apnea and modulate sleep function. Several studies are being conducted and should display breakthrough results soon.

References

[1] Franco, C. M., Lima, A. M., Ataíde, L. Jr, Lins, O. G., Castro, C. M., Bezerra, A. A., de Oliveira, M. F., Oliveira, J. R. Obstructive sleep

apnea severity correlates with cellular and plasma oxidative stress parameters and affective symptoms. *J. Mol. Neurosci.* 2012 Jun;47(2): 300-10. doi: 10.1007/s12031-012-9738-0.

[2] Cao, J., Feng, J., Li, L., Chen, B. Obstructive sleep apnea promotes cancer development and progression: a concise review. *Sleep Breath.* 2015 Feb. 3.

[3] Yaranov, D. M., Smyrlis, A., Usatii, N., Butler, A., Petrini, J. R., Mendez, J., Warshofsky, M. K. Effect of obstructive sleep apnea on frequency of stroke in patients with atrial fibrillation. *Am. J. Cardiol.* 2015 Feb. 15;115(4):461-5. doi: 10.1016/j.amjcard.2014.11.027. Epub. 2014 Nov. 29.

[4] de Oliveira, M. F., Pinto, F. C., Rotta, J. M. Normal pressure hydrocephalus in a professional athlete: a model of brain functional reserve. *J. Neuropsychiatry Clin. Neurosci.* 1;26(2):E39-40, 2014.

[5] Hanigan, W. C., Zallek, S. N. Headaches, shunts, and obstructive sleep apnea: report of two cases. *Neurosurgery.* 2004 Mar;54(3):764-8; discussion 768-9.

[6] Jennum, P., Borgesen, S. Intracranial pressure and obstructive sleep. *Chest* 95:279-83, 1989.

[7] Krauss, J. K., Droste, D. W., Bohus, M., Regel, J. P., Scheremet, R., Riemann, D., Seeger, W. The relation of intracranial pressure B-waves to different sleep stages in patients with suspected normal pressure hydrocephalus. *Acta Neurochir.* (Wien) 136(3-4):195-203, 1995.

[8] Kristensen, B., Malm, J., Rabben, T. Effects of transient and persistent cerebrospinal fluid drainage on sleep disordered breathing in patients with idiopathic adult hydrocephalus syndrome. *J. Neurol. Neurosurg. Psychiatry* 65(4):497-501, 1998.

[9] Kuchiwaki, H., Misu, N., Hirai, N., et al. Pre- and postoperative studies of sleep levels in patients with normal pressure hydrocephalus for an indication of operative treatment. In: Dietz, H., Brock, M., Klinger, M., ed. *Advances in neurosurgery.* Berlin: Springer-Verlag, 13:296-303s, 1985.

[10] McNamara, M. E., Millman, R. P., Epstein, M. H., Fogel, B. S. The association of normal-pressure hydrocephalus with obstructive sleep apnea. *J. Geriatr. Psychiatry Neurol.* 5(4):238-40, 1992.

[11] Newell, D. W., Aaslid, R., Stoos, R., et al. The relationship of blood flow velocity fluctuations to intracranial pressure B-waves. *J. Neurosurg.* 76:415-21, 1992.

[12] Oliveira, M. F., Oliveira, J. R., Rotta, J. M., Pinto, F. C. Psychiatric symptoms are present in most of the patients with idiopathic normal pressure hydrocephalus. *Arq. Neuropsiquiatr*. 72(6):435-8, 2014.

[13] Botelho, R. V., Bittencourt, L. R., Rotta, J. M., Tufik, S.: A prospective controlled study of sleep respiratory events in patients with craniovertebral junction malformation. *J. Neurosurg*. 99:1004-1009, 2003.

[14] Botelho, R. V., Bittencourt, L. R., Rotta, J. M., Tufik, S. Polysomnographic respiratory findings in patients with Arnold-Chiari type I malformation and basilar invagination, with or without syringomyelia: preliminary report of a series of cases. *Neurosurg. Rev*. 2000 Sep;23(3):151-5.

[15] Losurdo, A., Dittoni, S., Testani, E., Di Blasi, C., Scarano, E., Mariotti, P., Paternoster, G., Di Rocco, C., Massimi, L., Della Marca, G. Sleep disordered breathing in children and adolescents with Chiari malformation type I. *J. Clin. Sleep Med*. 2013 Apr. 15;9(4):371-7. doi: 10.5664/jcsm.2592.

[16] Luigetti, M., Losurdo, A., Dittoni, S., Testani, E., Colicchio, S., Gnoni, V., Farina, B., Scarano, E., Zampino, G., Mariotti, P., Rendeli, C., Di Rocco, C., Massimi, L., Della Marca, G. Improvement of obstructive sleep apneas caused by hydrocephalus associated with Chiari malformation Type II following surgery. *J. Neurosurg. Pediatr*. 2010 Oct;6(4):336-9. doi: 10.3171/2010.7.PEDS10207.

[17] Botelho, R. V., Bittencourt, L. R., Rotta, J. M., Tufik, S. Adult Chiari malformation and sleep apnoea. *Neurosurg. Rev*. 2005 Jul;28(3):169-76. Epub. 2005 May 21.

[18] Massimiliano, V., Della Pepa, G. M., Giuseppe, B., Aldo, S. Reversible and delayed isolated central sleep apnea after cervical laminectomy: report of the first case. *Acta Neurochir*. (Wien). 2014 Feb;156(2):267-8. doi: 10.1007/s00701-013-1904-9. Epub. 2013 Oct. 30.

[19] Naim-Ur-Rahman. Post-operative central sleep apnoea complicating cervical laminectomy: case report. *Br. J. Neurosurg*. 1994;8(5):621-5.

[20] Eyigor, H., Selcuk, O. T., Osma, U., Koca, R., Yilmaz, M. D. Cervical osteophytes: a rare cause of obstructive sleep apnea. *J. Craniofac. Surg*. 2012 Sep;23(5):e444-6. doi: 10.1097/SCS.0b013e318260e9ea.

[21] Khan, A., Than, K. D., Chen, K. S., Wang, A. C., La Marca, F., Park, P. Sleep apnea and cervical spine pathology. *Eur. Spine J*. 2014 Mar;23(3): 641-7. doi: 10.1007/s00586-013-3046-4. Epub. 2013 Oct. 9.

[22] Della Pepa, G. M., La Rocca, G., Barbagallo, G., Spallone, A., Visocchi, M. Transient breathing disorders after posterior cervical surgery for degenerative diseases: pathophysiological interpretation. *Eur. Rev. Med. Pharmacol. Sci.* 2014;18(1 Suppl.):89-92.

[23] Chen, J. C., Hwang, J. H. Sleep apnea increased incidence of primary central nervous system cancers: a nationwide cohort study. *Sleep Med.* 2014 Jul;15(7):749-54. doi: 10.1016/j.sleep.2013.11.782. Epub. 2014 Mar. 24.

[24] Pulcherio, J. O., Velasco, C. M., Machado, R. S., Souza, W. N., Menezes, D. R. Forestier's disease and its implications in otolaryngology: literature review. *Braz. J. Otorhinolaryngol.* 2014 Apr; 80(2):161-6.

[25] Erol, F. S., Kaplan, M. Spontaneous pneumocephalus presenting with apnea attacks in a newborn with open myelomeningocele. *Pediatr. Neurosurg.* 2004 Nov-Dec;40(6):312-3.

[26] Leduc, B. E., Dagher, J. H., Mayer, P., Bellemare, F., Lepage, Y. Estimated prevalence of obstructive sleep apnea-hypopnea syndrome after cervical cord injury. *Arch. Phys. Med. Rehabil.* 2007 Mar;88(3): 333-7.

[27] Raslan, A. M. Percutaneous computed tomography-guided transdiscal low cervical cordotomy for cancer pain as a method to avoid sleep apnea. *Stereotact. Funct. Neurosurg.* 2005;83(4):159-64. Epub. 2005 Oct. 17.

[28] Welt, S., Maurer, J. T., Hörmann, K., Stuck, B. A. Radiofrequency surgery of the tongue base in the treatment of snoring--a pilot study. *Sleep Breath.* 2007 Mar;11(1):39-43.

[29] Zaidi, F. N., Meadows, P., Jacobowitz, O., Davidson, T. M. Tongue anatomy and physiology, the scientific basis for a novel targeted neurostimulation system designed for the treatment of obstructive sleep apnea. *Neuromodulation.* 2013 Jul-Aug;16(4):376-86; discussion 386. doi: 10.1111/j.1525-1403.2012.00514.x.

[30] Horner, R. L. Neuromodulation of hypoglossal motoneurons during sleep. *Respir. Physiol. Neurobiol.* 2008 Dec. 10;164(1-2):179-96. doi: 10.1016/j.resp.2008.06.012.

In: Obstructive and Central Sleep Apnea
Editor: Joan McCormick
ISBN: 978-1-63483-335-6

Chapter 4

Changes in the Eye Related to Obstructive Sleep Apnea Syndrome

Blanca Ferrandez[1], MD, Pilar Calvo[1], MD, PhD, and Antonio Ferreras[1,2], MD, PhD

[1] Department of Ophtalmology. Miguel Servet University Hospital. Aragon Health Research Institute, IIS Aragón, Zaragoza, Spain

[2]University of Zaragoza, Spain

Abstract

Obstructive sleep apnea syndrome (OSAS) is defined by partial (hypopnea) or complete (apnea) intermittent episodes of upper airway collapse during sleep. The hypoxia resulting from these repetitive episodes leads to oxidative stress, sympathetic activation, endothelial dysfunction, systemic inflammation, and metabolic abnormalities. These pathophysiologic mechanisms are the source of many systemic diseases, such as blood and pulmonary hypertension, insulin resistance, metabolic syndrome, arrhythmia, myocardial infarction, congestive heart failure, and stroke. OSAS affects approximately 24% of men and 9% of women in the general population, and its prevalence increases with age. Different ophthalmologic disorders are also associated with OSAS: floppy eyelid syndrome, retinal vein occlusion, primary open angle glaucoma, normal-tension glaucoma, papilledema, non-ischemic anterior optic neuropathy, and central serous retinopathy. Changes in the optic nerve head (ONH) and retinal nerve fiber layer (RNFL) thickness in patients with OSAS have been a topic of controversy in recent years. Some studies have hypothesized that the hypoxia resulting from apnea-hypopnea episodes could compromise ONH vascularization. This condition may produce retinal ganglion cell damage and, consequently, reduce RFNL thickness. Some investigators report that OSAS and its severity could be related to decreased RNFL thickness or reduced retinal sensitivity measured with standard automated perimetry. On the other hand, other studies found no evidence of a correlation between OSAS and RFNL thickness loss. Different study designs, methodology, inclusion and exclusion criteria, age, and level of OSAS make it difficult to compare the results among several studies.

Thus, the structural and functional changes in the retina and optic disc due to OSAS remain unclear. Further prospective longitudinal studies are needed to elucidate the effect of OSAS on the eye.

Introduction

Obstructive sleep apnea syndrome (OSAS) is a chronic disorder characterized by total (apnea) or partial (hypopnea) upper airway collapse during sleep. Apnea is defined as a greater than 90% reduction in airflow lasting more than 10 seconds, and hypopnea is defined as a 30% to 90% reduction in airflow lasting more than 10 seconds in association with at least 3% arterial blood oxygen desaturation. This situation results in intermittent hypoxia, micro-arousals, and sleep fragmentation. When the apnea/hypopnea index (AHI) is at least five events per hour, OSAS is considered a clinical disorder. OSAS is a public health problem, not only for its high prevalence, but also due to its comorbidity. Young et al. [1] estimated that the prevalence of sleep-disorder breathing, defined as five events (apnea-hypopnea) per hour was 24% in men and 9% in women in the general population. Extrapolating to the general population, the authors estimated that 2% of female and 4% of middle-aged male active workers meet the minimum criteria for a diagnosis of OSAS. The prevalence increases with age, reaching as high as 33% to 77% among the obese population and diabetics [2]. OSAS is associated with a poor quality of life [3], motor vehicle accidents [4], depression and anxiety [5], memory problems, and attention and concentration defects [6]. Sympathetic activation, oxidative stress, and systemic inflammation, consequences of the apnea-hypopnea episodes, cause cardiovascular, neurologic, and endocrine diseases [7-15] in association with OSAS.

The severity of OSAS is classified as mild, moderate, and severe, depending on the AHI. The AHI is the total number of apneic and hypoapneic episodes per hour. Mild OSAS is defined as an AHI between 5 and 15, moderate OSAS is defined as an AHI > 15 and < 30, and severe OSAS is defined as an AHI > 30.

OSAS is diagnosed based on night-time polysomnography, which includes electroencephalography, electromyography, electrocardiography, respiratory movements, and pulse oximetry measurements, along with other measures [16, 17]. Clinical prediction equations to determine the sleep apnea clinical score allow for increased diagnostic efficiency.

Weight control is the most important general treatment measure and applicable in all patients. A 10% decrease in the body mass index can reduce the AHI by as much as 20% [18]. OSAS patients should not smoke or drink alcohol, and should avoid sedatives [19-21].

Some mechanical devices can be applied to produce positive pressure in the airway. These devices work by increasing the transmural pressure (positive transmural pressure), extending the pharynx area, increasing the lung volume, and preventing collapse [22-23]. There are three main types of devices: Continuous positive airway pressure devices apply new technology that automatically titrates positive airway pressure (APAP) [24] and bilevel positive airway pressure (BiPAP) [25].

Ophthalmologic Manifestations of OSAS

OSAS is associated with numerous systemic disorders, including ophthalmic pathology. Floppy eyelid syndrome (FES), glaucoma, nonarteritic anterior ischemic optic neuropathy, and papilledema are the most frequent ophthalmic pathologies associated with OSAS.

FES is the ocular pathology most commonly associated with OSAS and was initially described by Culbertson and Ostler in 1981 [26]. The prevalence of FES in OSAS patients is estimated to range from 2.3% to 32.6% depending on the study [27-29]. In FES, the upper eyelid is hyperlax, which facilitates its eversion. This condition causes the eye surface to be exposed, which may lead to unilateral or bilateral chronic papillary conjunctivitis, itching, and ocular irritation [30]. FES is more common in young patients and those with severe

OSAS[28]. Conservative treatment, such as lubrication or night occlusion can be effective in some cases, but other patients require surgical treatment for the eyelid hyperlaxity [31].

Primary open angle glaucoma is a multifactorial, progressive optic neuropathy and it is the most common form of glaucoma. This chronic neuropathy is characterized by the neurodegeneration of retinal ganglion cells, which leads to changes in the optic nerve head (ONH) and the retinal nerve fiber layer (RNFL), and visual field (VF) loss [32]. Glaucoma is the fourth leading cause of irreversible blindness in the world and the second cause of vision loss in people over 40 years in the Western world [33]. High intraocular pressure (IOP) is the main risk factor for developing glaucoma [34], but is not the only one. Other theories suggest the importance of adequate vascularization of the ONH in the pathogenesis of glaucoma [35]. The estimated prevalence of glaucoma in white populations ranges from 0.4% to 1.6% between 40 and 65 years, and increases to 6% in those older than 70 years [36]. Some studies show a higher rate of association between glaucoma and OSAS than in the general population [37-41]. Awareness of these findings will enhance the management and screening of vascular risk factors that can aggravate glaucoma optic neuropathy in these patients.

Some studies have demonstrated an association between OSAS and normal-tension glaucoma (NTG) [42-44]. NTG is an open angle glaucoma (open anterior chamber angle on gonioscopy) with characteristic VF defects and a maximum IOP below 21mm Hg. The prevalence of NTG is higher in women [45] and increases with age, from ~0.2% in the 43 to 54-year age group to 1.6% in those over 75 years of age [46]. NTG is associated with vasospastic disorders, systemic hypotension, and migraines. Although the pathogenesis of NTG is unclear, the cause of the ONH damage is possibly secondary to a chronic progressive ischemic disorder with hypoperfusion [47]. These disorders, such as chronic ischemia and hypoperfusion of the ONH, can occur in the context of OSAS as they are closely related entities.

Non-arteritic anterior ischemic optic neuropathy (NAION) is the most common acute neuropathy in patients over 50 years. It is caused by a circulatory disorder in the posterior ciliary arteries that nourish the optic nerve. Clinically, it is characterized by unilateral and painless loss of vision upon awakening in the morning, which is usually irreversible. Eye examination frequently reveals a relative afferent pupillary defect, optic disc edema, dyschromatopsia, and altitudinal VF loss [48]. It is associated with nocturnal systemic hypotension in patients with cardiovascular risk factors such as atherosclerosis and hypertension [47]. The prevalence of OSAS is higher in patients with NAION [47, 50, 51]. In fact, 70% to 80% of patients with NAION have OSAS. Why NAION occurs in OSAS patients is unclear, but it has been hypothesized that apnea episodes might lead to acute increases in blood pressure, intracranial pressure (ICP), or nocturnal hypoxemia, which could cause optic nerve edema and ischemia [51]. Although it is not possible to reverse vision loss from NAION, treatment for OSAS may help prevent an attack of NAION in the other eye, which occurs in 15% to 18% of cases.

Papilledema is swelling of the ONH caused by an increase in the ICP. The ICP increase causes papilledema due to the obstruction of retrograde axonal transport at the optic disc. Studies in animals and humans suggest that hypercapnia can induce cerebral vasodilation, which may be the main underlying mechanism of the nocturnal ICP increase in OSAS patients [52, 53]. Basic treatment of papilledema secondary to OSAS is continuous positive airway pressure.

Other less prevalent ophthalmologic disorders are also reported in patients affected by OSAS. Retinal vein occlusion (RVO) is one of the most common retinal vascular disorders and can have similar pathophysiologic mechanisms as OSAS. Both entities share risk factors, such as hypertension, diabetes mellitus, hyperlipidemia, and coronary artery disease. OSAS is associated with deep vein thrombosis and pulmonary embolism. Some studies indicate that individuals with OSAS have a higher prevalence of RVO and sleep apnea is an independent risk factor for RVO [54-56]. Central serous retinopathy is a serous neurosensory retinal detachment more common in middle-aged men and it is a rare ocular disorder associated with OSAS. Some studies report increased corticosteroid and catecholamine levels in central serous retinopathy, and sympathetic activity could be increased in OSAS, depending on the severity [57].

Study of the Retinal Fiber Layer in OSAS

Recent studies investigated the relationship between OSAS and RNFL thickness. The majority of these studies examined whether OSAS patients have RFNL damage associated with chronic and intermittent hypoxia.

The RNFL is formed mainly by retinal ganglion cell axons. Damage to retinal ganglion cells causes irreversible neuronal death that results in vision loss. Axonal damage can be detected and quantified by recently developed ocular imagining technologies, such as optical coherence tomography (OCT) and Scanning laser polarimetry (SLP).

OCT allows for examination of the posterior and anterior eye at an extremely fine spatial scale, without surgical biopsy or even any contact with the eye. OCT has objective and reproducible parameters that provide quantitative RNFL measurements and is the most commonly used imaging technology for examination of the ONH. Spectral domain (SD) OCT, such as the Cirrus OCT (Carl Zeiss Meditec, Dublin, CA) and Spectralis OCT (Heidelberg Engineering, Heidelberg, Germany), are faster and provide higher-quality images than the previous time domain (TD) OCT (Stratus OCT, Carl Zeiss Meditec, Dublin, CA). Cirrus SD-OCT acquires OCT data about 70 times faster (27,000 vs. 400 A-scans per second) and with better resolution (5 μm vs. 10 μm axial resolution in tissue), compared to first-generation OCT technology. Spectralis OCT integrates OCT with confocal scanning laser ophthalmoscopy and includes active eye tracking and noise reduction to improve the images.

SLP is a confocal scanning laser ophthalmoscope based on the principle that polarized light passing through the birefringent RNFL undergoes a measurable phase shift, known as retardation, which is linearly related to RNFL tissue thickness [58]. The cornea also exhibits birefringent properties, which are significantly neutralized in SLP with variable corneal compensation (VCC) [59]. The latest generation of SLP, SLP with enhanced corneal compensation (ECC), includes an enhancement module to improve the performance of SLP-VCC for detection of RNFL damage and progressive RNFL changes [60].

The pathogenesis of neurodegeneration due to OSAS is not completely clear. There are three main mechanisms of damage: intermittent hypoxemia-reoxygenation, changes in intrathoracic pressure during episodes of apnea and hypopnea, and micro-arousals [61]. The hypoxemia- reoxygenation cycles that occur during the night cause vascular endothelium damage, which produces inflammation-promoting substances [62], such as C-reactive protein, tumor necrosis factor [63-65], and interleukins. In addition, coagulation factors are activated [66, 67], leading to increased blood viscosity and platelet aggregation [68]. In the reoxygenation periods, reactive oxidant species are liberated, producing oxidative stress [69].

These phenomena can compromise normal vascularization and perfusion of the ONH. The blood supply from the posterior ciliary arteries to the short posterior ciliary arteries may be altered, decreasing perfusion of the anterior part of the ONH and neuronal ischemia. In glaucoma, neuropathy may similarly occur according to Anderson's vascular theory [70] that ischemia and alterations in the microcirculation could interfere with axonal nutrition and axoplasmic flow, leading to ONH damage.

Studies of RFNL and OSAS have produced different results. Comparison of the results of these studies is difficult, however, due to the use of different methods to measure RFNL thickness, different study populations, and different study designs.

Kargi et al. [71] and Moghimi et al. [72] measured RNFL thickness with SLP. Both studies reported decreased RNFL thickness in OSA patients. Kargi et al. reported that the majority of RNFL parameters were reduced in OSAS patients compared with healthy subjects. Moreover, they reported a strong correlation between AHI and reduced RNFL thickness. Moghimi et al. found a statistically significant difference between the two groups in disk average, superior average, and nerve fiber indicator. They did not, however, find correlations between the severity of the apnea (AHI) and RNFL thickness measurements. There was only a small but significant correlation between AHI and nerve fiber indicator. Both studies used previous versions of the GDx (Kargi et al. used the GDx FCC and Moghimi et al. used the GDx VCC) for RFNL measurements. This could be a limitation because measurements obtained using these GDx versions vary and are not as accurate as those obtained using the GDx ECC or spectral domain OCT. Moreover, Moghimi et al. did not exclude patients with glaucoma, which could be another limitation of their study.

Lin et al. [73] compared RNFL thickness, ONH parameters, and macular thickness between OSAS patients and a control group. Using the Stratus OCT to evaluate the RNFL and macular thickness, they found that the RNFL thickness measurements in the average and superior quadrant were significantly lower in the severe OSAS group compared to the control and mild OSAS groups. AHI and RNFL thickness, however, were not significantly correlated. In addition, they found no significant differences between groups in VF obtained with the Swedish interactive threshold algorithm (SITA) standard 30-2 Humphrey automated perimetry (Carl Zeiss Meditec Inc., Dublin, CA, USA). Further, macular thickness measurements did not differ significantly among the mild, moderate, and severe OSAS groups and controls.

Casas et al. [74] and Sagiv et al. [75] used the Stratus OCT to measure peripapillary RFNL thickness. They did not perform a VF test. Sagiv et al. demonstrated differences in average RNFL thickness between controls and OSAS patients. The RNFL thickness of the superior, inferior, and temporal quadrants was significantly reduced in the study group compared to the OSAS group. Casas et al. only found a significant decrease in RFNL thickness in the nasal quadrant in the OSAS group. A study by Adam et al. [76] of RFNL thickness in OSAS patients using the Stratus OCT and a VF test performed with the Humphrey Field Analyzer 750i SITA standard 30-2 revealed no significant differences between groups in RFNL thickness or VF. TD OCT technology has worse scan resolution and a slower scanning rate than the SD OCT [77] so this could be a limitation for studies using the Stratus OCT.

Huseyinoglu et al. [78] investigated 101 patients with OSAS and 20 controls. They studied RFNL thickness, ganglion cell complex (GCC) thickness in the macular region, and VF. OCT was performed using the RTVue version 4.0 (Optovue, USA) and VF examination was performed using the Octopus 900 (Haag-Streit International, Koeniz, Switzerland) perimeter. They found significant differences in the RNFL and GCC thickness values. Both RFNL and GCC thickness were lower in the severe OSAS group compared to the other groups. Pattern standard deviation values were significantly higher in all OSAS subgroups compared to the control group, and MD values were significantly lower in all OSAS patients compared to the control group.

Ferrandez et al. studied 80 OSAS patients and 111 age-matched controls [79]. RFNL thickness was measured with SD OCT and at least one reliable standard automated perimetry test was performed (24-2 SITA Standard algorithm). OSAS patients were classified into three groups based on the AHI: mild, moderate, or severe. Patients with glaucomatous SAP defects, glaucomatous optic disc morphology, or IOP > 20 mm Hg were excluded. Peripapillary RNFL thickness was measured using the Optic Disc Cube 200 x 200 acquisition protocol of the OCT device (Cirrus HD, software version 6.2; Carl Zeiss Meditec, Dublin, CA, USA). The main SAP indices differed significantly between groups. Mean deviation (MD) and the visual field index were lower in the OSAS group compared to the control group and pattern standard deviation was higher in the OSAS group. Most of the VF threshold values at each of the 52 VF points tested by the grid of the 24-2 SITA Standard strategy were depressed in OSAS patients compared with the control group. RNFL thickness measured with OCT did not differ significantly between groups. A limitation of this study, however, is that the control group did not undergo an overnight sleep study. It was assumed that the control group had no apnea/hypopnea events per hour based on the inclusion and exclusion criteria.

Discussion

The neurodegenerative mechanisms in OSAS patients are not completely clear. Most analyses of the ONH in OSAS patients suggest that intermittent nocturnal hypoxia and hypercapnia maintained over time is the main cause of ONH damage. Intermittent hypoxia produces endothelial injury that leads to the production of reactive oxygen species and inflammatory cytokines [57], such as interleukin-6 and 8, tumor necrosis factor α, and C reactive protein. Vascular coagulation is also altered during the hypoxemia episodes. Animal studies indicate that reactive oxygen species released during the reoxygenation periods have deleterious effects on the body, such as decreased ventricular function [80] and decreased nitric oxide bioavailability [81], which induce apoptosis in cortical neurons [82] and could be related to daytime sleepiness [83]. These mechanisms are all potential causes of the progressive loss of optic nerve fibers.

Some investigators have examined neurodegeneration in OSAS patients using functional studies such as neurocognitive tests, and structural studies such as single-photon emission-computed tomography, magnetic resonance spectroscopy, and cerebral blood flow to detect brain atrophy related to OSAS [84]. In the same way, OCT may be used as a structural test to study the neurodegeneration associated with OSAS.

OCT provides an accessible window for studies of the central nervous system. The retina contains unmyelinated axons that exit the ganglion cells of retina and are a unique part of the commissure of the superior colliculum. OCT can be useful for diagnosing and monitoring other systemic disorders that can affect the ONH, such as Parkinson disease, multiple sclerosis, and Alzheimer's disease [85-87]. In the same way, OCT could be used to analyze the possible neurodegeneration produced by OSAS.

One issue to consider is the difference between NTG and optic nerve degeneration caused by the OSAS mechanism. Both entities share more or less the same pathophysiologic mechanisms and may not be easy to distinguish. NTG is related to vascular factors such as abnormal ocular blood flow, systemic hypotension, coagulation alteration, ischemic vascular disorders, autoimmune disorders, migraines, and Raynaud's phenomenon. Some studies indicate that the prevalence of NTG in OSAS patients is higher than that in the general population and OSAS is a risk factor for NTG [42]. It remains unclear, however, whether ONH damage in OSAS patients, which has been reported in different studies, is produced in the context of NTG or whether it is caused by

OSAS independent of NTG. If it is independent of NTG and the ONH damage is produced by persistent hypoxemia and hypercapnia, alterations of the ONH could serve as a biomarker of neurodegeneration in OSAS patients.

OCT allows for quantitative and reproducible measurements of RNFL thickness and measurements of the progressive degeneration of ganglion cell axons. Extrapolation of studies of the ONH to the rest of the central nervous system may provide clues to other changes at the neuronal level. Therefore, OCT may be useful for follow-up studies of neurodegenerative processes due to OSAS.

Some studies indicate that ONH injury is not reflected by RFNL thickness measured by OCT, but VF defects may be detected [79]. Ferrandez et al. demonstrated that retinal sensitivity is reduced in OSAS patients compared with healthy subjects. Future studies should assess the use objective functional tests, such as electrophysiology. Thus, the role of VF in the evaluation of the neurodegeneration of OSAS remains unclear, but it may contribute to assessments of retinal damage in these patients.

Other multicenter and prospective studies with a greater number of patients are needed to continue this line of research offering a new perspective for follow-up of OSAS. Findings published to date provide promising results as a foundation for future studies.

References

[1] Duran-Cantalloa J. et al. Consenso nacional sobre el síndrome de apneas-hipopneas del sueño (SAHS). *Grupo español del sueño (GES).* Sept 2005.

[2] Young T, Palta M, Dempsey J, Skatrud J, Weber S, Badr S. The occurrence of sleep-disordered breathing among middle-aged adults. *N Engl J Med.* 1993 Apr 29;328(17):1230-5.

[3] Young T, Peppard PE, Taheri S. Excess weight and sleep disordered breathing. *J Appl Physiol* 2005;99:1592-9.

[4] Lacasse Y, Godbout C, Sériès F. Health-related quality of life in obstructive sleep apnoea. *Eur Respir J* 2002;19:499-503.

[5] Mulgrew AT, Nasvadi G, Butt A, et ál. Risk and severity of motor vehicle crashes in patients with obstructive sleep apnoea/hypopnoea. *Thorax* 2008; 63:536-541.

[6] Sharafkhaneh A, Giray N, Richardson P, Young T, Hirshkowitz M. Association of psychiatric disorders and sleep apnea in a large cohort. *Sleep* 2005;28:1405 1411.

[7] Landis CA. Neural activation patterns during working memory tasks and OSA disease severity: preliminary findings. *J Clin Sleep Med* 2009;5:21-27.

[8] Lavie P, Ben-Yosef R, Rubin AE. Prevalence of sleep apnea syndrome among patients with essential hypertension. *Am Heart J* 1984;108:373-376.

[9] Tsai JC. Neurological and neurobehavioral sequelae of obstructive sleep apnea. *Neuro Rehabilitation.* 2010;26:85–94.

[10] Hung J, Whitford EG, Parsons RW, Hillman DR. Association of sleep apnoea with myocardial infarction in men. *Lancet* 1990;336:261-264.

[11] Aurora RN, Punjabi NM. Obstructive sleep apnoea and type 2 diabetes mellitus: a bidirectional association. *Lancet Respir Med.* 2013;1:329–338.

[12] Guilleminault C, Connolly SJ, Winkle RA. Cardiac arrhythmia and conduction disturbances during sleep in 400 patients with sleep apnea syndrome. *Am J Cardiol* 1983;52:490-494.

[13] Surani SR. Diabetes, sleep apnea, obesity and cardiovascular disease: Why not address them together? *World J Diabetes*. 2014;5:381–384.

[14] Malone S, Liu PP, Holloway R, Rutherford R, Xie A, Bradley TD. Obstructive sleep apnea in patients with dilated cardiomyopathy: effects of continuous positive airway pressure. *Lancet* 1991;338:1480-1484.

[15] Weitzenblum E, Krieger J, Apprill M, et ál. Daytime pulmonary hypertension in patients with obstructive sleep apnea syndrome. *Am Rev Respir Dis* 1988;138:345-349.

[16] Palomäki H, Partinen M, Erkinjuntti T, Kaste M. Snoring, sleep apnea syndrome, and stroke. *Neurology* 1992;42(7 Suppl 6):75-82.

[17] Kushida CA, Littner MR, Morgenthaler T, et ál. Practice parameters for the indications for polysomnography and related procedures: an update for 2005. *Sleep* 2005;4:499-519.

[18] Ross SD, Sheinhait IA,Harrison KJ, et ál. Systematic review and meta-analysis of the literature regarding the diagnosis of sleep apnea. *Sleep* 2000;23:519-532.

[19] Peppard PE, Young T, Palta M, Dempsey J, Skatrud J. Longitudinal study of moderate weight change and sleep-disordered breathing. *JAMA* 2000;284:3015-3021.

[20] Wetter DW, Young TB, Bidwell TR, Badr MS, Palta M. Smoking as a risk factor for sleep-disordered breathing. *Arch Intern Med* 1994;154:2219-2224.

[21] Scanlan MF, Roebuck T, Little PJ, Redman JR, Naughton MT. Effect of moderate alcohol upon obstructive sleep apnoea. *Eur Respir J* 2000;16: 909-913.

[22] Mendelson WB, Garnett D, Gillin JC. Flurazepam-induced sleep apnea syndrome in a patient with insomnia and mild sleep-related respiratory changes. *J Nerv Ment Dis* 1981;169:261-264.

[23] Kakkar RK, Berry RB. Positive airway pressure treatment for obstructive sleep apnea. *Chest* 2007;132:1057-1072.

[24] Sullivan CE, Issa FG, Berthon-Jones M, Eves L. Reversal of obstructive sleep apnoea by continuous positive airway pressure applied through the nares. *Lance*t 1981;1:862-865.

[25] Littner M, Hirshkowitz M, Davila D, Anderson WM, Kushida CA, Woodson BT, Johnson SF, Merrill SW; Standards of Practice Committee of the American Academy of Sleep Medicine. Practice parameters for the use of auto-titrating continuous positive airway pressure devices for titrating pressures and treating adult patients with obstructive sleep apnea syndrome. An American Academy of Sleep Medicine report. *Sleep.* 2002 Mar 15;25(2):143-7.

[26] Resta O, Guido P, Picca V, et ál. Prescription of nCPAP and nBIPAP in obstructive sleep apnoea syndrome: Italian experience in 105 subjects. A prospective two centre study. *Respir Med* 1998;92:820-827.

[27] Culbertson WW, Ostler HB. The floppy eyelid syndrome. *Am J Ophthalmol.* 1981;4:568-75.

[28] McNab AA. Floppy eyelid syndrome and obstructive sleep apnea. *Ophthal Plast Reconstr Surg.* 1997;13:98-114.

[29] Mojon DS, Goldblum D, Fleischhauer J, Chiou AG,Frueh BE, Hess CW, et al. Eyelid, conjunctival, and corneal findings in sleep apnea syndrome. *Ophthalmology.* 1999;106:1182-5.

[30] Karger RA, White WA, Park WC, Rosales AG, McLaren JW, Olson EJ, et al. Prevalence of floppy eyelid syndrome in obstructive sleep apnea-hypopnea syndrome. *Ophthalmology.* 2006;113:1669-74.

[31] McNab AA. Floppy eyelid syndrome and obstructive sleep apnea. *Ophthal Plast Reconstr Surg.* 1997 Jun;13(2):98-114.

[32] Miyamoto C, Espírito Santo LC, Roisman L, Moreno Pde A, Cariello AJ, Osaki MH. Floppy eyelid syndrome: review. *Arq Bras Oftalmol.* 2011 Jan-Feb;74(1):64-6.

[33] Kroese M, Burton H, Vardy S, Rimme T, McCarter D. Prevalence of primary open angle glaucoma in general ophthalmic practice in the United Kingdom. *Br J Ophthalmol* 2002;86:978-80.

[34] American Academy of Ophthalmology Glaucoma Panel. Preferred Practice Pattern. Primary open-angle glaucoma. San Francisco, CA: *American Academy of Ophthalmology*; 2005:3.

[35] Anderson DR. Glaucoma, capillaries and pericytes. 1. Blood flow *regulation. Ophthalmologica.* 1996;210:257–262.

[36] Rudnicka AR, Mt-Isa S, Owen CG, Cook DG. Ashby D. Variations in primary open-angle glaucoma prevalence by age, gender, and race: A Bayesian meta-analysis. IOVS 2006;47:4254-61. Allingham R.R., Damji K., Freedman S., Moroi S. Shields' Textbook of Glaucoma. Philadelphia: *Williams & Wilkins; 2004.*

[37] Mojon DS, Hess CW, Goldblum D, et al. Primary open-angle glaucoma is associated with sleep apnea syndrome. *Ophthalmologica* 2000;214:115—8.

[38] Onen SH, Mouriaux F, Berramdane L, et al. High prevalence of sleep-disordered breathing in patients with primary open-angle glaucoma. *Acta Ophthalmol Scand* 2000;78:638—41.

[39] Hashim SP, Al Mansouri FA, Farouk M, Al Hashemi AA, Singh R. Prevalence of glaucoma in patients with moderate to severe obstructive sleep apnea: ocular morbidity and outcomes in a 3 year follow-up study. *Eye* (Lond) 2014;28(11):1304-9.

[40] Balbay EG, Balbay O, Annakkaya AN, Suner KO, Yuksel H, Tunç M, Arbak P. Obstructive sleep apnoea syndrome in patients with primary open-angle glaucoma. *Hong Kong Med J* 2014;20(5):379-85.

[41] Pérez-Rico C, Gutiérrez-Díaz E, Mencía-Gutiérrez E, Díaz-de-Atauri MJ, Blanco R. Obstructive sleep apnea-hypopnea syndrome (OSAHS) and glaucomatous optic neuropathy. *Graefes Arch Clin Exp Ophthalmol* 2014;252(9):1345-57.

[42] Sergi M, Salerno DE, Rizzi M, Blini M, Andreoli A, Messenio D, Pecis M, Bertoni G. Prevalence of normal tension glaucoma in obstructive sleep apnea syndrome patients. *J Glaucoma.* 2007 Jan;16(1):42-6.

[43] Mojon DS, Hess CW, Golbdlum D, et al. Normal-tension glaucoma is associated with sleep apnea syndrome. *Ophthalmologica.* 2002; 216:180–184.

[44] Marcus DM, Costarides AP, Gokhale P, et al. Sleep disorders: a risk factor for normal-tension glaucoma? *J Glaucoma.* 2001;10:177–183.

[45] Levene R. Low tension glaucoma: a critical review and new material. *Surv Ophthalmol*. 1980;61:621–664.
[46] Klein B, Klein R, Sponsel WE, et al. Prevalence of glaucoma: the Beaver Dam Eye Study. *Ophthalmology*. 1992;99:1499–1504.
[47] Hayreh SS, Zimmerman MB, Podhajsky P, et al. Nocturnal arterial hypotension and its role in optic nerve head and ocular ischemic disorders. *Am J Ophthalmol.* 1994;117:603–624.
[48] Rizzo JF, 3rd, Lessell S. Optic neuritis and ischemic optic neuropathy. Overlapping clinical profiles. *Arch Ophthalmol. Dec* 1991; 109(12):1668-1672.
[49] Bilgin G, Koban Y, Arnold AC. Nonarteritic anterior ischemic optic neuropathy and obstructive sleep apnea. *J Neuroophthalmol.* 2013 Sep;33(3):232-4.
[50] Mojon DS, Hedges TR, 3rd, Ehrenberg B, et al. Association between sleep apnea syndrome and nonarteritic anterior ischemic optic neuropathy. *Arch Ophthalmol.* May 2002;120(5):601-605.
[51] Li J, McGwin G, Jr., Vaphiades MS, Owsley C. Non-arteritic anterior ischaemic optic neuropathy and presumed sleep apnoea syndrome screened by the Sleep Apnea scale of the Sleep Disorders Questionnaire (SA-SDQ). *Br J Ophthalmol.* Nov 2007;91(11):1524-1527.
[52] Sugita YIijima STeshima Y et al. Marked episodic elevation of cerebrospinal fluid pressure during nocturnal sleep in patients with sleep apnea hypersomnia syndrome. *Electroencephalogr Clin Neurophysiol.* 1985;60214- 219.
[53] Purvin VA, Kawasaki A, Yee RD. Papilledema and obstructive sleep apnea syndrome. *Arch Ophthalmol*. 2000 Dec;118(12):1626-30.
[54] Govetto A, Domínguez R, Rojas L, Pereiro M, Lorente R. Bilateral and simultaneous central retinal vein occlusion in a patient with obstructive sleep apnea syndrome. *Case Rep Ophthalmol.* 2014 May 21;5(2):150-6.
[55] Leroux les Jardins G, Glacet-Bernard A, Lasry S, Housset B, Coscas G, Soubrane G. Retinal vein occlusion and obstructive sleep apnea syndrome. *J Fr Ophtalmol.* 2009 Jun;32(6):420-4.
[56] Chou KT, Huang CC, Tsai DC, Chen YM, Perng DW, Shiao GM, Lee YC, Leu HB. Sleep apnea and risk of retinal vein occlusion: a nationwide population-based study of Taiwanese. *Am J Ophthalmol.* 2012 Jul;154(1):200-205.
[57] Kloos P, Laube I, Thoelen A. Obstructive sleep apnea in patients with central serous chorioretinopathy. *Graefes Arch Clin Exp Ophthalmol.* 2008 Sep;246(9).

[58] Weinreb RN, Shakiba S, Zangwill L. Scanning laser polarimetry to measure the nerve fiber layer of normal and glaucomatous eyes. *Am J Ophthalmol* 1995;119:627-636.
[59] Zhou Q, Weinreb RN. Individualized compensation of anterior segment birefringence during scanning laser polarimetry. *Invest Ophthalmol Vis Sci* 2002;43:2221-2228.
[60] Medeiros FA, Zangwill LM, Alencar LM, Sample PA, Weinreb RN. Rates of progressive retinal nerve fiber layer loss in glaucoma measured by scanning laser polarimetry. *Am J Ophthalmol* 2010;149:908–915.
[61] Torre-Bouscoulet L, Meza-Cargas MS, Castorena-Maldonado A, Pérez-Padilla R. Riesgo cardiovascular en adultos con síndrome de apnea obstructiva del sueño. A 25 años de los primeros estudios de asociación. *Gac Méd Mex* 2008;144:323-332.
[62] Ryan S, Taylor CT, McNicholas WT. Selective activation of inflammatory pathways by intermittent hypoxia in obstructive sleep apnea syndrome. *Circulation* 2005;112:2660-2667.
[63] Shamsuzzaman AS, Winnicki M, Lanfranchi P, et ál. Elevated C-reactive protein in patients with obstructive sleep apnea. *Circulation* 2002;105:2462-2464.
[64] Tauman R, Ivanenko A, O´Brien LM, Gozal D. Plasma C-reactive protein levels among children with sleepdisordered breathing. *Pediatrics* 2004; 113:e564-e569.
[65] Minoguchi K, Tazaki T, Yokoe T, et ál. Elevated production of tumor necrosis factor-alpha by monocytes in patients with obstructive sleep apnea syndrome. *Chest* 2004;126:1473-1479.
[66] Robinson GV, Pepperell JC, Segal HC, Davies RJ, Stradling JR. Circulating cardiovascular risk factors in obstructive sleep apnoea: data from randomized controlled trials. *Thorax* 2004;59:777-782.
[67] Shitrit D, Peled N, Shitrit AB, et ál. An association between oxygen desaturation and D-dimer in patients with obstructive sleep apnea syndrome. *Thromb Haemost* 2005;94:544-547.
[68] Steiner S, Jax T, Evers S, Hennersdorf M, Schwalen A, Strauer BE. Altered blood rheology in obstructive sleep apnea as a mediator of cardiovascular risk. *Cardiology* 2005;104:92-96.
[69] Dyugovskaya L, Lavie P, Lavie L. Increased adhesion molecules expression and production of reactive oxygen species in leukocytes of sleep apnea patients. *Am J Respir Crit Care Med* 2002;165:934-939.
[70] Anderson DR. Glaucoma, capillaries and pericytes. 1. Blood flow regulation. *Ophthalmologica.* 1996;210:257–262.

[71] Kargi SH, Altin R, Koksal M, et al. Retinal nerve fiber layer measurements are reduced in patients with obstructive sleep apnea syndrome. *Eye.* 2005;19:575–579.

[72] Moghimi S, Ahmadraji A, Sotoodeh H, et al. Retinal nerve fiber thickness is reduced in sleep apnea syndrome. *Sleep Med.*2013;14:53–57.

[73] Lin PW, Friedman M, Lin HC, Chang HW, Pulver TM, Chin CH. Decreased retinal nerve fiber layer thickness in patients with obstructive sleep apnea/hypopnea syndrome. *Graefes Arch Clin Exp Ophthalmol.* 2011;249:585–593.

[74] Casas P, Ascaso FJ, Vicente E, Tejero-Garces G, Adiego MI,Cristobal JA. Retinal and optic nerve evaluation by optical coherence tomography in adults with obstructive sleep apnea-hypopnea syndrome (OSAHS). *Graefes Arch Clin Exp Ophthalmol.* 2013;251:1625–1634.

[75] Sagiv O, Fishelson-Arev T, Buckman G, et al. Retinal nerve fiber layer thickness measurements by optical coherence tomography in patients with sleep apnea syndrome. *Clin Experiment Ophthalmol.* 2014;42:132–138.

[76] Adam M, Okka M, Yosunkaya S, Bozkurt B, Kerimoğlu H, Turan M. The evaluation of retinal nerve fiber layer thickness in patients with obstructive sleep apnea syndrome. *J Ophthalmol.* 2013;2013:292158.

[77] Chen TC, Cense B, Pierce MC, et al. Spectral domain optical coherence tomography: ultra-high speed, ultra-high resolution ophthalmic imaging. *Arch Ophthalmol.* 2005; 123:1715–20.

[78] Huseyinoglu N, Ekinci M, Ozben S, Buyukuysal C, Kale MY, Sanivar HS. Optic disc and retinal nerve fiber layer parameters as indicators of neurodegenerative brain changes in patients with obstructive sleep apnea syndrome. *Sleep Breath.* 2014;18:95–102.

[79] Ferrandez B, Ferreras A, Calvo P, Abadia B, Fogagnolo P, Wang Y, Marin JM, Iester M. Retinal sensitivity is reduced in patients with obstructive sleep apnea. *Invest Ophthalmol Vis Sci.* 2014 Oct 9;55(11):7119-25.

[80] Chen L, Einbinder E, Zhang Q, Hasday J, Balke CW, Scharf SM. Oxidative stress and left ventricular function with chronic intermittent hypoxia in rats. *Am J Respir Crit Care Med* 2005;172:915-920.

[81] Lavie L, Vishnevsky A, Lavie P. Evidence for lipid peroxidation in obstructive sleep apnea. *Sleep* 2004;27:123-128.

[82] Xu W, Chi L, Row BW, et ál. Increased oxidative stress is associated with chronic intermittent hypoxia-mediated brain cortical neuronal cell

apoptosis in a mouse model of sleep apnea. *Neuroscience* 2004;126:313-323.

[83] Veasey SC, Davis CW, Fenik P, et ál. Long-term intermittent hypoxia in mice: protracted hypersomnolence with oxidative injury to sleep-wake brain regions. *Sleep* 2004;27:194-201.

[84] Nowak M, Kornhuber J, Meyrer R (2006) Daytime impairment and neurodegeneration in OSAS. *Sleep* 29:1521–1530.

[85] Tian T, Zhu XH, Liu YH. Potential role of retina as a biomarker for progression of Parkinson's disease. *Int J Ophthalmol.* 2011;4:433–438.

[86] Fjeldstad AS, Carlson NG, Rose JW. Optical coherence tomography as a biomarker in multiple sclerosis. *Expert Opin Med Diagn*. 2012;6:593–604.

[87] Kesler A, Vakhapova V, Korczyn AD, Naftaliev E, Neudorfer M. Retinal thickness in patients with mild cognitive impairment and Alzheimer's disease. *Clin Neurol Neurosurg.* 2011;113: 523–526.

In: Obstructive and Central Sleep Apnea
Editor: Joan McCormick
ISBN: 978-1-63483-335-6

Chapter 5

QT Dispersion in Patients with Obstructive Sleep Apnea

Igor A. Kelmanson*
Institute of Special Education and Special Psychology of the Raoul Wallenberg International University for Family and Child, St. Petersburg, Russia

Abstract

Exaggerated dispersion of repolarization is likely to play a role in both the initiation and the maintenance of malignant ventricular arrhythmias. Inter-lead QT interval differences within a 12-lead ECG termed "QT dispersion" may reflect regional differences in myocardial refractoriness. QT dispersion is simply defined as the difference between the longest (QTmax) and the shortest (QTmin) QT intervals within a 12-lead ECG. Since the QT interval on its own may vary according to the heart rate, it may be corrected using Bazett's formula ($QT/\sqrt{RR}$) to give rise to QTc intervals, and the difference between QTcmax and QTcmin is the QTc dispersion (heart rate-corrected QT dispersion, QTcd). It has been supposed that one of the causes of the disturbed repolarization might be linked with autonomic imbalance, in that a decreased parasympathetic innervation exposes the heart to unopposed

* E-mail: iakelmanson@hotmail.com

stimulation by sympathetic nerves. This assuming, abnormal QT dispersion may be related to obstructive sleep apnea syndrome (OSAS). A meta-analysis encompassing 222 patients with diagnosed OSAS and 182 control subjects found higher values of QT dispersion in OSAS patients. Another finding was more prominent increase in QT dispersion in the female OSAS patients. The reasons may be significantly longer values of QTd and QTcd found in healthy men. These normally higher values may explain why the OSAS in male patients resulted in less effect compared with women. Increased QT dispersion in OSAS patients may reflect disturbed myocardial repolarization and predispose to cardiac arrhythmias.

Keywords: Arrhythmias, meta-analysis, obstructive sleep apnea, QT dispersion, repolarization

Introduction

Exaggerated dispersion of repolarization is likely to play a role in both the initiation and the maintenance of malignant ventricular arrhythmias by generating a substrate for functional re-entry (Issa, Miller, & Zipes, 2012; Saksena & Camm, 2012). It was proposed that the inter-lead QT interval differences within a 12-lead ECG might reflect regional differences in myocardial refractoriness, and that this might predict cardiac dysrhythmias. This range of the QT durations was termed "QT dispersion" (Day, McComb, & Campbell, 1990). It was proposed that the different ECG leads magnify the ECG signal of different myocardial regions and that, consequently, QT dispersion is an almost direct measure of the heterogeneity of myocardial repolarization (Malik & Batchvarov, 2000). Animal (Zabel, Portnoy, & Franz, 1995), and human (Zabel, Lichtlen, Haverich, & Franz, 1998) studies supported this hypothesis.

QT dispersion is simply defined as the difference between the longest (QTmax) and the shortest (QTmin) QT intervals within a 12-lead ECG. Since the QT interval on its own may vary according to the heart rate, it may be corrected using Bazett's formula ($QT/\sqrt{RR}$) to give rise to QTc intervals, and the difference between QTcmax and QTcmin is the QTc dispersion (heart rate-corrected QT dispersion, QTcd).

The average normal value of QT dispersion in normal subjects was ≤ 40 ms in 13 studies and ≥ 40 ms in eight studies (Surawicz, 1996). Perhaps the

QT dispersion in normal subjects should be ≤ 50 ms (Statters, Malik, Ward, & Camm, 1994).

Abnormal repolarization featuring as increased QT dispersion is known to contribute to the fatal mechanisms associated with numerous cardiovascular pathologies (Barr, Naas, Freeman, Lang, & Struthers, 1994; Cin, Celik, & Ulucan, 1997; Galinier et al., 1997; Galinier et al., 1998). Disturbances of repolarization were also found in patients with certain psychopathological conditions, particularly with anxiety spectrum disorders (Kelmanson, 2014a).

It has been supposed that one of the causes of the disturbed repolarization might be linked with autonomic imbalance, in that a decreased parasympathetic innervation exposes the heart to unopposed stimulation by sympathetic nerves (Saksena & Camm, 2012), and it has been shown that sympathetic hyperactivity, specifically an imbalance between left and right stellate ganglion activity, promotes a prolonged and increased dispersion of repolarization, thereby lowering the ventricular fibrillation threshold (Schwartz, 1985).

Particular attention was paid to the effects of sleep disordered breathing on the autonomic function during sleep and wake states. Sleep disordered breathing refers to a range of pathological conditions characterized by abnormal respiratory function during sleep. The most common manifestation of sleep disordered breathing is apnea (cessation of airflow) or hypopnea (a reduction in ventilation) and depending on the severity, result in varying degrees of hypoxia, hypercapnia, and fragmented sleep. Obstructive sleep apnea (OSA) is the most common form of apnea and is the most frequent reason for referral to a sleep disorders laboratory for formal evaluation by overnight polysomnography.

Individuals with OSA may stop breathing many times during the night due to repeated apneas or hypopneas arising from airway obstruction. The autonomic response to apneas and hypopneas is a complex sequence of events leading to sympathetic activation involving multiple mechanisms including peripheral and central chemoreceptor stimulation (Lanfranchi & Somers, 2011). It has been suggested that the two main determinants of the heart rate variability changes in OSA are an alteration of central cardiac–respiratory coupling, which is significantly impaired in OSA; and an attenuation of the baroreflexes, compared to normal subjects (Jo et al., 2005). The hemodynamic alterations in OSA patients during the apneic episodes are a strong indicator of the cardiovascular "storm" that is associated with each apneic event. Normally, lung inflation inhibits the sympathetic activity. However, during apnea, this mechanism is lacking, thereby leading to a marked sympathetic activation resulting in acute cardiovascular effects, such as a marked elevation in the blood pressure and bradycardic/tachycardic events (Somers et al., 2008). The apneic events are also associated with an increased sympathetic modulation (Kelmanson, 2014b; Kesek, Franklin, Sahlin, & Lindberg, 2009; Park et al., 2008). This sympathetic overdrive is highest when hypoxemia and hypercapnia reach maximal levels at the end of an apnea. The subsequent airway reopening is associated with a large increase in the blood pressure, primarily due to the synergistic effect of the peripheral vasoconstriction, increased venous return and thus cardiac output. The arterial pressure rise activates the baroreflex control mechanisms, thereby inducing a temporary shutdown of the sympathetic over-activity (Narkiewicz & Somers, 2001). Based on these findings, some authors suggested that variations in heart rate during breathing may serve as a screening method for OSA (Guilleminault, Connolly, Winkle, Melvin, & Tilkian, 1984; Penzel, Glos, Schobel, Lal, & Fietze, 2013).

Meanwhile, the studies examining QT dispersion in patients with OSA are relatively scarce, and the numbers of patients that entered these studies were limited.

A meta-analysis covering the period from 2000 through 2014 was performed aimed at the identification of the relevant studies (Kelmanson, 2015). Four studies that compared QT dispersion values in subjects with OSA and in the controls were identified. Table 1 is the summary of these papers. Overall, these studies encompassed 222 patients with diagnosed OSA (168 male, 54 female) and 182 control subjects (109 male, 73 female). Three studies (Dursunoglu et al., 2005; Khositseth, Nantarakchaikul, Kuptanon, & Preutthipan, 2011; Nakamura et al., 2004) encompassing 178 OSA patients (134 male, 44 female) and 144 control subjects (84 male, 60 female) were performed on the adult population, while one study (Khositseth, et al., 2011) that included 44 OSA patients (34 boys, 10 girls) and 38 controls (25 boys, 13 girls) was performed on children. Mean calculated age of the OSA patients across all the studies was 37,7 years (standard error 11.5 years). Mean calculated age of the OSA patients in the studies covering adult patients was 45.7 years (standard error 0.7 years).

Table 2 summarises raw data on QT dispersion values extracted from the studies. In two studies (Dursunoglu, et al., 2005; Khositseth, et al., 2011), the values of QT dispersions (either crude or heart rate-corrected) were statistically significantly higher in the patients from the OSA group compared with controls. In one study where the comparisons were separately performed in the male and female patients (Voigt, Haq, Mitre, Lombardo, & Kassotis,

2011), the values of QT dispersions (either crude or heart rate-corrected) were statistically significantly higher in the female patients from the OSA group compared with controls, while the differences in male subgroup were insignificnat. In one study (Nakamura, et al., 2004) the differences between groups were insignificant.

Crude QT dispersion values were available in 193 patients with diagnosed OSA and in 162 controls. Heart-rate-corrected QT dispersion values were available in 191 patients with diagnosed OSA and in 182 controls. The summary of the meta-anaysis of the values of the standardized mean differences calculated as Hedges's g for crude and heart-rate-corrected QT dispersions estimates are provided on Figure 1. In two of three studies, the values of crude QT dispersion were statistically significantly higher in patients with diagnosed OSA. The values of crude and rate-corrected QT dispersions in the OSA groups exceeded 50 ms, which is considered as the upper normal limit (Statters, et al., 1994). Aggregated standardised difference in the means was equal to 0.571 (95% CI: 0.354 – 0.789; SE = 0.111, $p < 0.001$). In three of four studies, the values of heart-rate-corrected QT dispersion were significantly higher in patients with diagnosed OSA. Aggregated standardised difference in the means was equal to 0.859 (95% CI: 0.142 – 1.577; SE = 0.366, $p = 0.019$).

Looking at the point-estimates of the aggregate standardised differences in the means calcualated for the crude (QTd) and heart-rate-corrected (QTcd) dispersions, the first impression was that the effect size of OSA is more prominent for the values of QTcd. However, 95% confidence interval around the point estimate of the aggregate standardised differences in the means of QTcd was wider than around the ones of QTd, and the confidence intervals were overlapping. Therefore, there is no reason to speak of any stitistically significant differences between the effect sizes as measured by these two different approaches. This is in accord with the opinion of some authors who have expressed their skepticism about the need to correct QT for the heart rate (Kautzner, Yi, Camm, & Malik, 1994; Malik & Camm, 1997). The estimated values of the aggregate standardized effect sizes (Hedges's g) for the crude and rate-corrected QT dispersions may be characterized as medium to large (as has been determined, the medium effect sizes correspond to Hedges's values $\geq$ 0.5, while large to values $\geq$ 0.8 (Cohen, 1988)). Substantial variations in the calculated effect sizes of OSA on QTd and QTcd raised the question whether these variations are exceptionally due to within-study error or may partly reflect variations in the true effects. There was reason to believe that the effect might have been influenced by several moderating factors. Among possible candidates were the mean ages of the patients from the OSA groups, proportions of the male subjects in these groups and the mean values of the obstructive AHI in the certain OSA groups that entered the analysis. To test this hypothesis, a meta-regression analysis was performed, in that potential moderators were entered into the model as the predictors. Mixed-effect model (method of moments) was used (Borenstein, Hedges, Higgins, & Rothstein, 2005). No statistically significant association was found between the effect sizes on the one hand (calculated either as QTd or QTcd) and the values of the mean age of the patients who entered the OSA groups. The studies were further categorized as either performed in the adults or in the children, and the age group category was added as another moderator. This enabled to run a separate analysis for each level of the age group and to compare the effects at different levels of this category. Again, no statistically significant difference was found between the subgroups for the values of the effect sizes. No statistically significant association was found between the values of the effect size and the reported mean values of the AHI in the OSA group. Meanwhile, statistically significant association was found between the effect sizes estimated as QTd and the proportion of male patients in the OSA group (intercept = 1.40, regression coefficient = - 0.011, $p = 0.0003$) (Figure 2). As it comes from the plot, the effect size decreased with growing percent of male patients in the OSA sample. Similar trend was found for the effect sizes estimated as QTcd, although in that case the association failed to reach the level of statistical significance (intercept = 1.84, regression coefficient = - 0.015, $p = 0.061$).

Chronic intermittent hypoxemia following repetitive apneic episodes and cyclic disruption of the sleep architecture caused by the arousals induce a complex series of both acute and chronic changes. The chronic consequences primarily involve the baroreflex and chemoreflex control mechanisms, with a higher sympathetic modulation and a blunted parasympathetic control of heart rate variability (Smith, Veale, Pepin, & Levy, 1998). An autonomic profile characterized by sympathetic predominance was suggested by the studies comparing OSA with control subjects (Kesek, et al., 2009; Narkiewicz & Somers, 2003; Parish & Somers, 2004; Smietanowski, Szelenberger, & Trzebski, 2006; Vanninen, Tuunainen, Kansanen, Uusitupa, & Lansimies, 1996). A meta-analysis found the evidence on increased sympathetic tone on children with diagnosed OSA with statistically significant positive association between the reported values of the mean obstructive AHI and the degree of increased sympathetic tone (Kelmanson, 2014b). Such autonomic imbalance may lead to disturbed myocardial repolarization manifesting as increased QT dispersion. It was found that increased QTd was positively correlated with increased sympathetic and/or decreased vagal modulations (Ishida et al., 1997). It has been shown that QTd is a significant predictor of cardiovascular mortality (Okin et al., 2000). OSA is associated with increased cardiovascular morbidity such as hypertension, ischemic heart disease, congestive heart failure, cardiac arrhythmias, cerebrovascular disease and cardiovascular mortality (McNicholas, Bonsigore, & Management Committee of, 2007; Somers, et al., 2008), and it has been hypothesized that sympathetic activation plays an important role in these risks (Narkiewicz & Somers, 2001).

The ECG recordings, which QT dispersions have been measured, were performed in the wake state. One could suppose that the autonomic disturbances resulted from OSA could have manifested at most during sleep time. However, OSA subjects may have a sympathetic overdrive even during wakefulness, when the abnormal breathing pattern and the altered blood gas exchange observed during sleep cannot be acutely responsible for the hemodynamic and autonomic alterations (Narkiewicz et al., 1998; Somers, Dyken, Clary, & Abboud, 1995). This increase may be unrelated to blood pressure values (Carlson et al., 1993). Some authors found that OSA in children was associated with a higher sympathetic activity during sleep and lower sympathetic level at daytime, thus leading them to a conclusion that short-term effect of OSA in the young patients may be more prominent than long-term one (Weller et al., 2006). Meanwhile, the findings were that disturbed repolarization in OSA patients featuring as increased QT dispersion on the surface ECG could be well identified during daytime, either in pediatric or in adult patients. This meta-analysis failed to find any age-related differences in the associations between OSA and QT dispersion on the surface ECG registered in the wake state.

Surprisingly, meta-analysis failed to find significant associations between the reported values of AHI in the OSA groups and the values of the standardized effect sizes of QT dispersion, as might have been expected. One explanation may be relative similarities of the reported values of AHI in the studies covered by the analysis: they varied between 42.4 and 51.9 events/hour. As well, the number of studies included into analysis was relatively small, which might be a source of a reduced statistical power.

A commonly used diagnostic criteria for OSA syndrome in adults has been set as AHI $\geq$ 5/hour associated with symptoms or an AHI $\geq$ 15/hour with or without associated symptoms; AHI equal to 5–15 events/hour usually identifies mild OSA, AHI 15–30 events/hour is moderate OSA and AHI > 30 events/hour is usually considered as severe OSA. Meanwhile, the diagnostic criteria of pediatric OSA are different, and most clinicians make the diagnosis of pediatric OSA based on an obstructive AHI greater than 1 to 2/hour (Berry, 2012). Obstructive AHI less than 5 events/hour is usually termed as mild, and AHI equal to 5 and more is considered as moderate-to-severe, as in the studies that entered this meta-analysis. However, it has been acknowledged that the cutoffs of these scores are largely arbitrary and some other criteria should be used to properly grade the severity of sleep disordered breathing (Spruyt, 2012). The repetitive apneic episodes that induce hypoxemia, hypercapnia and alterations of neural circulatory activation are responsible for an enhanced sympathetic drive (Jo, et al., 2005; Somers, et al., 2008), and this effect should be proportional to the number and durations of obstructive events. It seems likely that the signs of significantly deteriorated autonomic tone in patients with OSA may become evident, only when the frequency of obstructive events during sleep and the degree of physiological disturbances associated with these events will reach certain critical level. Sometimes moderate OSA cases in adult patients were characterized by clear sympathetic over-activity, while severe ones were associated with a lower sympathetic modulation (Gula et al., 2003; Kesek, et al., 2009).

Another interesting finding is negative association between the effect size of OSA on QT dispersion and the proportion of male subjects in the OSA groups across the studies included into this meta-analysis, meaning that the effect was more prominent in the females. Some authors reported that in an overtly healthy population of men and women, there was a change in QTd as a function of gender. Significantly longer values of QTd and QTcd were found in healthy men (Kassotis, Costeas, Bedi, Tolat, & Reiffel, 2000). This difference was explained by a longer QTc min found in women, and this longer QTc min was shown to increase their risk of developing drug induced life-threatening cardiac arrhythmia in women known as "torsades de pointes" (Makkar, Fromm, Steinman, Meissner, & Lehmann, 1993). The normally higher values of QTd and QTcd in men may explain why the OSA in male patients resulted in less effect size compared with women, although QTd and QTcd in both men and women with OSA appear to be higher when compared with a normal population. One should acknowledge that the measurement of the QT interval and its dispersion has not been standardized, and the studies are affected by fundamental limitations of the use of QTd (QTcd) measurements.

The accuracy of the QT interval and dispersion measurements have been limited by difficulties with reliable identification of T-wave offset (Zabel, et al., 1995). Nor the measurement of the OSA severity is strictly standardized so far.

Table 1. Studies included into meta-analysis (Kelmanson, 2015)

Source	Study and patients characteristics	Author-specified rules for the scoring of the respiratory events
Nakamura et al., 2004 (Nakamura, et al., 2004)	Forty-eight OSA patients (45 men, 3 women) without cardiac diseases (mean [±SD] age, 45.9 ± 10.8 years; apnea-hypopnea index [AHI] 51.9 ± 18.5 events per hour) who underwent polysomnography before treatment and on the first night of nasal continuous positive airway pressure (nCPAP) treatment. The measurements of QTcd after sleep were obtained and included into analysis. As a control, QTcd was also measured in the morning from 26 healthy subjects (24 men, 2 women).	The OSA patients underwent polysomnography. Apnea was defined as a complete cessation of airflow at the nose and mouth that lasts for ≥ 10 s. Hypopnea was defined as a decrease of ≥ 50% in thoracoabdominal motion that lasts for ≥ 10 s and is associated with a fall in the baseline SaO_2 of ≥ 4%. All AHI values were calculated to express the number of episodes of apnea and hypopnea per hour of total sleep time.
Dursunoglu et al., 2005 (Dursunoglu, et al., 2005)	A total of 49 subjects without hypertension, diabetes mellitus, any cardiac or pulmonary diseases, or any hormonal, hepatic, renal or electrolyte disorders were referred for evaluation of OSA. An overnight polysomnography and a standard 12-lead ECG were performed in each subject. According to the apnoea-hypopnoea index (AHI), subjects were divided into control subjects (AHI < 5, n = 20, 11 men, 9 women, age 45.0 ± 4.6 years) and moderate-severe OSA patients (AHI > or = 15, n = 29, 16 men, 13 women, age 45.8 ± 5.1 years).	An apnea was defined as total obstruction of oronasal airflow for ≥ 10 s, a hypopnea was defined as a decrease of airflow of ≥ 50% and desaturations were accepted as a ≥ 4% decrease in oxygen saturation. The desaturation index was identified as the number of oxygen desaturation events per hour of sleep. Subjects with an AHI ≥ 5 were diagnosed as OSA (Anonymous, 1999).
Khositseth et al., 2011 (Khositseth, et al., 2011)	Forty-four children (34 male) with OSA syndrome, aged 6.2 ± 3.5 years along with 38 healthy children (25 male), aged 6.6 ± 2.1 years, underwent electrocardiography to measure QT and RR intervals. The authors excluded children with conditions or diseases that may interfere with the QT interval including cardiac, pulmonary, renal, hepatic diseases, systemic hypertension, epilepsy, having a history of previous arrhythmia or palpitation, family history of sudden death in a younger age – less than 35 years – taking medications that may prolong the QT interval, and craniofacial malformation or major anomalies.	The diagnosis of OSA syndrome was made by either overnight polysomnography or overnight oximetry. The criterion for diagnosis of OSA syndrome by polysomnography was defined as mixed/obstructive apnea/ hypopnea index greater than or equal to 5 events per hour (American Thoracic Society, 1996). The diagnosis of obstructive sleep apnea syndrome by overnight oximetry was defined as a cluster of desaturation, five or more desaturations occurring in a 10- to 30-minute period (Brouillette et al., 2000).

Table 1. (Continued)

Source	Study and patients characteristics	Author-specified rules for the scoring of the respiratory events
Voigt et al., 2011 (Voigt, et al., 2011)	There were 199 patients studied: 73 men aged 45.4 ± 13.7 years and 28 women aged 45.3 ± 11.4 years with OSA diagnosed in sleep centre; and 49 men aged 55.5 ± 17.4 years and 49 women aged 54.4 ± 18.2 years without OSA from the ambulatory cervices, representing the control group. Patients with OSA had recorded objective sleep study parameters, including apnea-hypopnea index (AHI). QT intervals were measured in each of the 12 leads of a standard surface electrocardiogram during wakefulness; QTd and QTcd were calculated. Echocardiograms were obtained prior to recruitment in this study and patients with significant structural heart disease were excluded. Patients were also excluded if they had a history of coronary artery disease, were currently being treated for hypertension, were using psychotropic, cardiac medications, contraceptive pills or hormonal replacement therapy, and if they had any disorder or electrolyte imbalance known to affect the QT interval. Patients were also excluded if they had frequent ventricular ectopy during the sleep study.	Not specified

Table 2. Raw findings from the studies included into meta-analysis (Kelmanson, 2015)

Study name	Subgroup within study	Comparison	OSA mean (ms)	OSA standard deviation (ms)	OSA sample size	Control mean (ms)	Control standard deviation (ms)	Control sample size	P value
Nakamura et al., 2004	Blank	QTd	60.0	12.7	48	54.4	14.5	26	0.086
Nakamura et al., 2004	Blank	QTcd	60.5	12.5	48	59.6	16.1	26	0.794
Dursunoglu et al., 2005	Blank	QTcd	56.1	9.3	29	36.3	4.5	20	0.000
Khositseth et al., 2011	Blank	QTd	52.0	27.0	44	40.0	14.0	38	0.014
Khositseth et al., 2011	Blank	QTcd	71.0	29.0	44	57.0	19.0	38	0.011
Voigt et al., 2011	Men	QTd	56.0	35.0	73	48.0	19.0	49	0.144
Voigt et al., 2011	Men	QTcd	58.0	34.0	73	53.0	21.0	49	0.359
Voigt et al., 2011	Women	QTd	54.0	21.0	28	31.0	13.0	49	0.000
Voigt et al., 2011	Women	QTcd	58.0	22.0	28	34.0	15.0	49	0.000

Study name	Subgroup within study	Comparison	Statistics for each study		
			Hedges's g	Lower limit	Upper limit
Khositseth, 2011	Blank	QTd	0,541	0,103	0,979
Nakamura, 2004	Blank	QTd	0,414	-0,063	0,891
Voigt, 2011	Combined	QTd	0,645	0,350	0,939
			0,571	0,354	0,789

Hedges's g and 95% CI

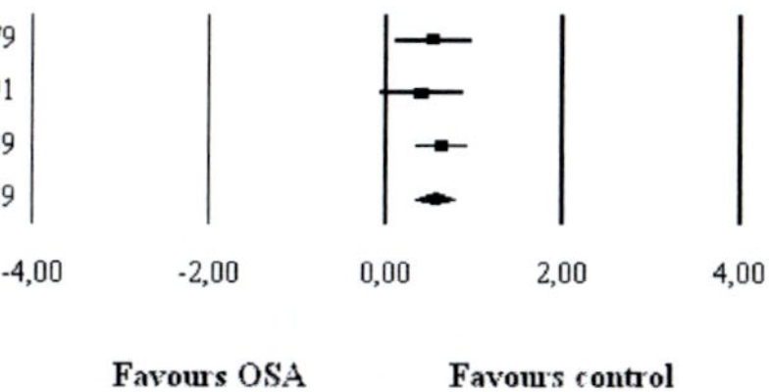

Meta-analysis of crude QT dispersion values

Study name	Subgroup within study	Comparison	Statistics for each study		
			Hedges's g	Lower limit	Upper limit
Dursunoglu, 2005	Blank	QTcd	2,521	1,771	3,272
Khositseth, 2011	Blank	QTcd	0,557	0,119	0,996
Nakamura, 2004	Blank	QTcd	0,063	-0,409	0,535
Voigt, 2011	Combined	QTcd	0,560	0,267	0,854
			0,859	0,142	1,577

Hedges's g and 95% CI

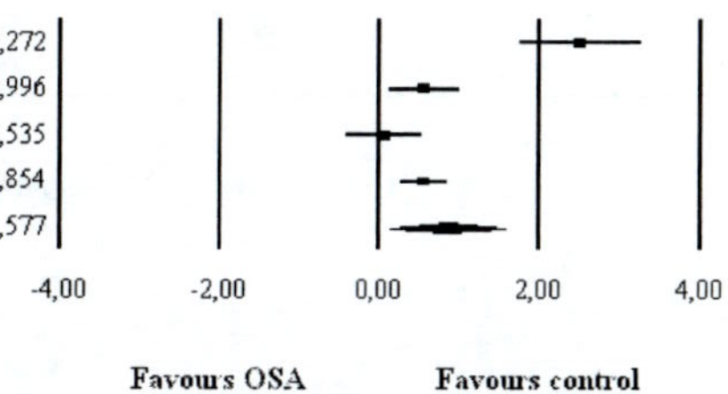

Figure 1. Meta-analysis of QT dispersion values (Kelmanson, 2015).

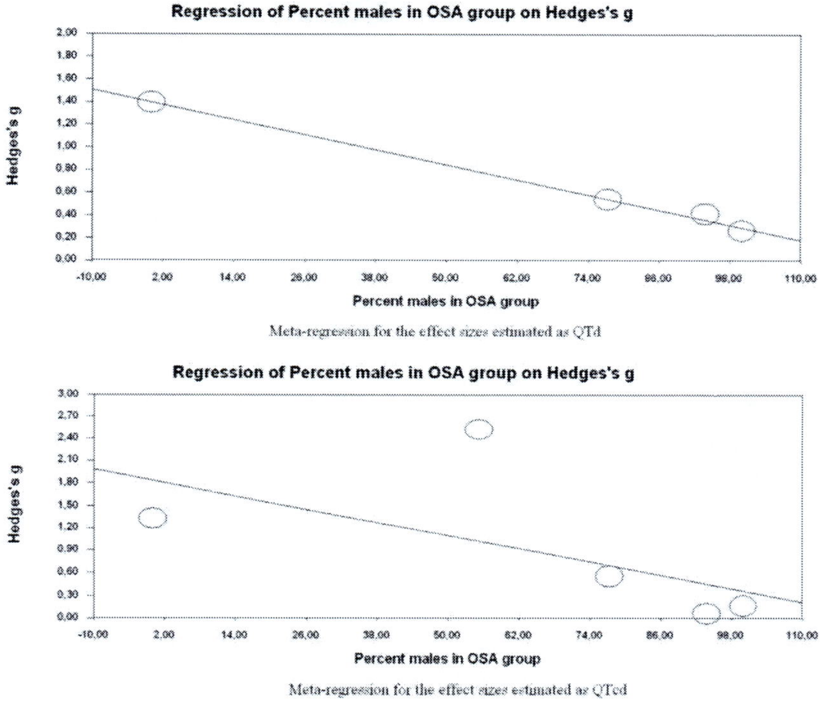

Figure 2. Meta-regression of the percent of male patients in the OSA group on Hedges's g values (Kelmanson, 2015).

Although most authors explicitly used the similar and generally approved criteria to the identification of the respiratory events during sleep, one should admit certain inevitable inconsistencies in the diagnosis of OSA. As well, marked changes in the severity of OSA between the nights may be noted, which may lead, in turn, to the underestimation of the respiratory events and mask sleep laboratory results (Spruyt, 2012).

With all limitations in mind, the findings are indicative that OSA is associated with increased QT dispersion. This may reflect disturbed myocardial repolarization in patients with OSA and predispose them to cardiac arrhythmias.

References

American Thoracic Society (1996). Standards and indications for cardiopulmonary sleep studies in children. *Am. J. Respir. Crit. Care Med., 153*(2), 866-878. doi: 10.1164/ajrccm.153.2.8564147

Anonymous (1999). Sleep-related breathing disorders in adults: recommendations for syndrome definition and measurement techniques in clinical research. The Report of an American Academy of Sleep Medicine Task Force. *Sleep, 22*(5), 667-689.

Barr, C. S., Naas, A., Freeman, M., Lang, C. C., & Struthers, A. D. (1994). QT dispersion and sudden unexpected death in chronic heart failure. *Lancet, 343*(8893), 327-329.

Berry, R. B. (2012). *Fundamentals of sleep medicine*. Philadelphia, PA: Elsevier/Saunders.

Borenstein, M., Hedges, L., Higgins, J., & Rothstein, H. (2005). *Comprehensive Meta-analysis Version 2*. Englewood, NJ: Biostat.

Brouillette, R. T., Morielli, A., Leimanis, A., Waters, K. A., Luciano, R., & Ducharme, F. M. (2000). Nocturnal pulse oximetry as an abbreviated testing modality for pediatric obstructive sleep apnea. *Pediatrics, 105*(2), 405-412.

Carlson, J. T., Hedner, J., Elam, M., Ejnell, H., Sellgren, J., & Wallin, B. G. (1993). Augmented resting sympathetic activity in awake patients with obstructive sleep apnea. *Chest, 103*(6), 1763-1768.

Cin, V. G., Celik, M., & Ulucan, S. (1997). QT dispersion ratio in patients with unstable angina pectoris (a new risk factor?). *Clin. Cardiol., 20*(6), 533-535.

Cohen, J. (1988). *Statistical power analysis for the behavioral sciences* (2nd ed.). Hillsdale, N.J.: L. Erlbaum Associates.

Day, C. P., McComb, J. M., & Campbell, R. W. (1990). QT dispersion: an indication of arrhythmia risk in patients with long QT intervals. *Br Heart J., 63*(6), 342-344.

Dursunoglu, D., Dursunoglu, N., Evrengul, H., Ozkurt, S., Kilic, M., Fisekci, F. (2005). QT interval dispersion in obstructive sleep apnoea syndrome patients without hypertension. *Eur. Respir. J., 25*(4), 677-681. doi: 10.1183/09031936.05.00067104

Galinier, M., Balanescu, S., Fourcade, J., Dorobantu, M., Boveda, S., Massabuau, P. (1997). Prognostic value of ventricular arrhythmias in systemic hypertension. *J. Hypertens, 15*(12 Pt 2), 1779-1783.

Galinier, M., Vialette, J. C., Fourcade, J., Cabrol, P., Dongay, B., Massabuau, P. (1998). QT interval dispersion as a predictor of arrhythmic events in congestive heart failure. Importance of aetiology. *Eur. Heart J., 19*(7), 1054-1062.

Guilleminault, C., Connolly, S., Winkle, R., Melvin, K., & Tilkian, A. (1984). Cyclical variation of the heart rate in sleep apnoea syndrome. Mechanisms, and usefulness of 24 h electrocardiography as a screening technique. *Lancet, 1*(8369), 126-131.

Gula, L. J., Krahn, A. D., Skanes, A., Ferguson, K. A., George, C., Yee, R. (2003). Heart rate variability in obstructive sleep apnea: a prospective study and frequency domain analysis. *Ann. Noninvasive Electrocardiol., 8*(2), 144-149.

Ishida, S., Nakagawa, M., Fujino, T., Yonemochi, H., Saikawa, T., & Ito, M. (1997). Circadian variation of QT interval dispersion: correlation with heart rate variability. *J. Electrocardiol., 30*, 205-210.

Issa, Z. F., Miller, J. M., & Zipes, D. P. (2012). *Clinical arrhythmology and electrophysiology: a companion to Braunwald's heart disease* (2nd ed.). Philadelphia, PA: Elseiver/Saunders.

Jo, J. A., Blasi, A., Valladares, E., Juarez, R., Baydur, A., & Khoo, M. C. (2005). Determinants of heart rate variability in obstructive sleep apnea syndrome during wakefulness and sleep. *Am J Physiol Heart Circ Physiol, 288*(3), H1103-1112. doi: 10.1152/ajpheart.01065.2003

Kassotis, J., Costeas, C., Bedi, A. K., Tolat, A., & Reiffel, J. (2000). Effects of aging and gender on QT dispersion in an overtly healthy population. *Pacing Clin. Electrophysiol., 23*(7), 1121-1126.

Kautzner, J., Yi, G., Camm, A. J., & Malik, M. (1994). Short- and long-term reproducibility of QT, QTc, and QT dispersion measurement in healthy subjects. *Pacing Clin. Electrophysiol, 17*(5 Pt 1), 928-937.

Kelmanson, I. A. (2014a). High anxiety in clinically healthy patients and increased QT dispersion: a meta-analysis. *Eur. J. Prev. Cardiol., 21*(12), 1568-1574. doi: 10.1177/2047487313501613

Kelmanson, I. A. (2014b). Signs of sympathetic dominance in sleep and wake based on spectral analysis of heart rate variability in children with obstructive sleep apnea. *Somnologie - Schlafforschung und Schlafmedizin, 18*(3), 194-201. doi: 10.1007/s11818-014-0672-y

Kelmanson, I. A. (2015). Obstructive sleep apnea and increased QT-dispersion: a meta-analysis. *Somnologie - Schlafforschung und Schlafmedizin, 19*(4) (in press).

Kesek, M., Franklin, K. A., Sahlin, C., & Lindberg, E. (2009). Heart rate variability during sleep and sleep apnoea in a population based study of 387 women. *Clin Physiol Funct Imaging, 29*(4), 309-315. doi: 10.1111/j.1475-097X.2009.00873.x

Khositseth, A., Nantarakchaikul, P., Kuptanon, T., & Preutthipan, A. (2011). QT dispersion in childhood obstructive sleep apnoea syndrome. *Cardiol Young, 21*(2), 130-135. doi: 10.1017/S1047951110001514

Lanfranchi, P. A., & Somers, V. K. (2011). Cardiovascular physiology: Autonomic control in health and in sleep disorders. In M. H. Kryger, T. Roth & W. C. Dement (Eds.), *Principles and practice of sleep medicine* (5th ed., pp. 226-236). Philadelphia, PA: Saunders/Elsevier.

Makkar, R. R., Fromm, B. S., Steinman, R. T., Meissner, M. D., & Lehmann, M. H. (1993). Female gender as a risk factor for torsades de pointes associated with cardiovascular drugs. *JAMA, 270*(21), 2590-2597.

Malik, M., & Batchvarov, V. N. (2000). Measurement, interpretation and clinical potential of QT dispersion. *J. Am. Coll Cardiol., 36*(6), 1749-1766.

Malik, M., & Camm, A. J. (1997). Mystery of QTc interval dispersion. *Am. J. Cardiol., 79*(6), 785-787.

McNicholas, W. T., Bonsigore, M. R., & Management Committee of, E. C. A. B. (2007). Sleep apnoea as an independent risk factor for cardiovascular disease: current evidence, basic mechanisms and research priorities. *Eur Respir J, 29*(1), 156-178. doi: 10.1183/09031936.00027406

Nakamura, T., Chin, K., Hosokawa, R., Takahashi, K., Sumi, K., Ohi, M. (2004). Corrected QT dispersion and cardiac sympathetic function in patients with obstructive sleep apnea-hypopnea syndrome. *Chest, 125*(6), 2107-2114.

Narkiewicz, K., Montano, N., Cogliati, C., van de Borne, P. J., Dyken, M. E., & Somers, V. K. (1998). Altered cardiovascular variability in obstructive sleep apnea. *Circulation, 98*(11), 1071-1077.

Narkiewicz, K., & Somers, V. K. (2001). Cardiovascular variability characteristics in obstructive sleep apnea. *Auton Neurosci, 90*(1-2), 89-94. doi: 10.1016/S1566-0702(01)00272-7

Narkiewicz, K., & Somers, V. K. (2003). Sympathetic nerve activity in obstructive sleep apnoea. *Acta Physiol. Scand., 177*(3), 385-390. doi: 10.1046/j.1365-201X.2003.01091.x

Okin, P. M., Devereux, R. B., Howard, B. V., Fabsitz, R. R., Lee, E. T., & Welty, T. K. (2000). Assessment of QT interval and QT dispersion for prediction of all-cause and cardiovascular mortality in American Indians (The Strong Heart Study) *Circulation, 101*(1), 61-66.

Parish, J. M., & Somers, V. K. (2004). Obstructive sleep apnea and cardiovascular disease. *Mayo Clin Proc, 79*(8), 1036-1046. doi: 10.4065/79.8.1036

Park, D. H., Shin, C. J., Hong, S. C., Yu, J., Ryu, S. H., Kim, E. J. (2008). Correlation between the severity of obstructive sleep apnea and heart rate variability indices. *J. Korean Med. Sci., 23*(2), 226-231. doi: 10.3346/ jkms.2008.23.2.226

Penzel, T., Glos, M., Schobel, C., Lal, S., & Fietze, I. (2013). Estimating sleep disordered breathing based on heart rate analysis. *Conf Proc IEEE Eng Med Biol Soc, 2013*, 6571-6574. doi: 10.1109/EMBC.2013.6611061

Saksena, S., & Camm, A. J. (2012). *Electrophysiological disorders of the heart* (2nd ed.). Philadelphia: Elsevier/Saunders.

Schwartz, P. J. (1985). Idiopathic long QT syndrome: progress and questions. *Am. Heart J., 109*(2), 399-411.

Smietanowski, M., Szelenberger, W., & Trzebski, A. (2006). Nonlinear dynamics of the cardiovascular parameters in sleep and sleep apnea. In memory of Alberto Malliani (1935-2006)--a brave heart and beautiful mind. *J. Physiol. Pharmacol., 57 Suppl 11*, 55-68.

Smith, R. P., Veale, D., Pepin, J. L., & Levy, P. A. (1998). Obstructive sleep apnoea and the autonomic nervous system. *Sleep Med. Rev., 2*(2), 69-92.

Somers, V. K., Dyken, M. E., Clary, M. P., & Abboud, F. M. (1995). Sympathetic neural mechanisms in obstructive sleep apnea. *J. Clin. Invest., 96*(4), 1897-1904. doi: 10.1172/JCI118235

Somers, V. K., White, D. P., Amin, R., Abraham, W. T., Costa, F., Culebras, A. (2008). Sleep apnea and cardiovascular disease: an American Heart Association/American College of Cardiology Foundation Scientific Statement from the American Heart Association Council for High Blood Pressure Research Professional Education Committee, Council on Clinical Cardiology, Stroke Council, and Council on Cardiovascular Nursing. *J Am Coll Cardiol, 52*(8), 686-717. doi: 10.1016/j.jacc.2008.05.002

Spruyt, K. (2012). Pediatric sleep-disordered breathing: criteria and spectrum of disease. In L. Kheirandish-Gozal & D. Gozal (Eds.), *Sleep disordered breathing in children : a comprehensive clinical guide to evaluation and treatment* (pp. 245-260). New York: Humana Press.

Statters, D. J., Malik, M., Ward, D. E., & Camm, A. J. (1994). QT dispersion: problems of methodology and clinical significance. *J. Cardiovasc. Electrophysiol., 5*(8), 672-685.

Surawicz, B. (1996). Will QT dispersion play a role in clinical decision-making? *J. Cardiovasc. Electrophysiol., 7*(8), 777-784.

Vanninen, E., Tuunainen, A., Kansanen, M., Uusitupa, M., & Lansimies, E. (1996). Cardiac sympathovagal balance during sleep apnea episodes. *Clin. Physiol., 16*(3), 209-216.

Voigt, L., Haq, S. A., Mitre, C. A., Lombardo, G., & Kassotis, J. (2011). Effect of obstructive sleep apnea on QT dispersion: a potential mechanism of sudden cardiac death. *Cardiology, 118*(1), 68-73. doi: 10.1159/000324796

Weller, D., Paditz, E., Rüdiger, H., Hoyer, A., Schütze, P., & Scheuch, K. (2006). Veränderung der Herzfrequenzvariabilität, der Blutdruckvariabilität und der Baroreflexsensitivität tagsüber und im Schlaf bei Kindern mit obstruktivem Schlafapnoesyndrom. *Somnologie - Schlafforschung und Schlafmedizin, 10*(3), 130-137. doi: 10.1111/j.1439-054X.2006.00089.x

Zabel, M., Lichtlen, P. R., Haverich, A., & Franz, M. R. (1998). Comparison of ECG variables of dispersion of ventricular repolarization with direct myocardial repolarization measurements in the human heart. *J. Cardiovasc. Electrophysiol., 9*(12), 1279-1284.

Zabel, M., Portnoy, S., & Franz, M. R. (1995). Electrocardiographic indexes of dispersion of ventricular repolarization: an isolated heart validation study. *J. Am. Coll. Cardiol., 25*(3), 746-752. doi: 10.1016/0735-1097(94)00446-W.

Index

C

D

E

F

G

H

I

J

L

M

N

O

P

Q

R

S

T

U